Survival is the art of staying alive.

Mental attitude is as important as physical endurance and knowledge. You must know how to take everything possible from nature and use it to the fullest, how to attract attention to yourself so that rescuers may find you, and how to make your way across unknown territory back to civilization if there is no hope of rescue, navigating without map or compass. You must know how to maintain a healthy physical condition, or if sick or wounded, heal yourself and others. You must be able to maintain your morale and that of others who share your situation.

The Boy Scout's motto is the right one:

BE PREPARED!

HarperEssentials

CARD GAMES
FAMILY AND PARTY GAMES
FIRST AID
STRESS SURVIVAL GUIDE
THE ULTIMATE SURVIVAL GUIDE
UNDERSTANDING DREAMS
WINE GUIDE
YOGA
ZODIAC SIGNS

HARPERESSENTIALS

THE ULTIMATE SURVIVAL GUIDE

JOHN "LOFTY" WISEMAN

(Previously published as *SAS Survival Handbook*)

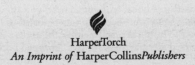

HarperTorch
An Imprint of HarperCollinsPublishers

This book was originally published as *SAS Survival Handbook* in 1986, then by HarperCollins UK in 1993 and 2004.

HARPERTORCH
An Imprint of HarperCollins*Publishers*
10 East 53rd Street
New York, New York 10022-5299

Copyright © John Wiseman 1986, 1993, 2004
Illustrations © HarperCollinsPublishers 1986, 1993
ISBN: 0-06-073434-5

First HarperTorch paperback printing: November 2004

Printed in the United States of America

Visit HarperTorch on the World Wide Web at www.harpercollins.com

10 9 8 7 6 5 4 3 2 1

WARNING

The survival techniques described in this publication are for use in dire circumstances where the safety of individuals is at risk. Accordingly the publishers cannot accept any responsibility for any prosecutions or proceedings brought or instituted against any person or body as a result of the use or misuse of any techniques described or any loss, injury or damage caused thereby. In practicing and perfecting these survival techniques the rights of landowners and all relevant laws protecting certain species of animals and plants and controlling the use of firearms and other weapons must be regarded as paramount.

CONTENTS

INTRODUCTION

FOR 26 years, as a professional soldier, I had the privilege to serve with the Special Air Service (SAS). This elite unit of the British Army is trained to carry out arduous operations in all parts of the world. They have to develop skills which enable them to survive anywhere and to handle every kind of situation. As survival instructor to the SAS it was my job to ensure that each and every member of the Regiment could apply these skills. Tested in training and operations, they form the basis of this book.

When I am teaching soldiers or civilians how to deal with survival situations, part of my job is to ensure their safety. I cannot do that for the reader of this book. I do know that what I have written has saved lives in the past and I can save more in the future. In learning the skills described here, readers must be restrained by the need to conserve our environment and to avoid cruelty to animals, and by-laws which some of these techniques may contravene. Remember, this is a handbook for the survival situation when self-preservation is paramount and risks may be involved which would otherwise be out of the question. You must apply survival techniques with caution, for the consequences will be your responsibility and no one else's.

Although this is not an official publication, by sharing survival knowledge gained through my SAS experience I aim to help you to be a survivor too.

J.W.
The Survival School, Hereford

ESSENTIALS
FOR SURVIVAL

SURVIVAL is the art of staying alive. Mental attitude is as important as physical endurance and knowledge. You must know how to take everything possible from nature and use it to the full, how to attract attention to yourself so that rescuers may find you, how to make your way across unknown territory back to civilization if there is no hope of rescue, navigating without map or compass. You must know how to maintain a healthy physical condition, or if sick or wounded heal yourself and others. You must be able to maintain your morale and that of others who share your situation.

Any equipment you have must be considered a bonus. Lack of equipment should not mean that you are unequipped, for you will carry skills and experience with you, but those skills and experience must not be allowed to get rusty and you must extend your knowledge all the time.

Think of survival skills as a pyramid, built on the foundation of the will to survive. The next layer of the pyramid is knowledge. It breeds confidence and dispels fears. The third layer is training: mastering skills and maintaining them. To cap the pyramid, add your kit. Combine the instinct for survival with knowledge, training and kit and you will be ready for anything.

BE PREPARED

The Boy Scouts' motto is the right one. Make sure you are physically and mentally prepared before you set out, and pack the appropriate gear for what you plan to do.

CHECK LIST

Before any journey or expedition ask yourself:

❑ How long will I be away?
❑ How much food and water do I need to carry?
❑ Have I the right clothing/footwear for the climate?
❑ Should I take standbys?
❑ What special equipment do I need for the terrain?
❑ What medical kit is appropriate?

HEALTH CHECKS

Have thorough medical and dental check-ups and ensure that you have all the necessary injections for the territories through which you intend to travel.

Pack a medical kit to cover all your likely needs and those of each member of your group.

GROUP EXPEDITIONS

Consider the ability of each member to deal with the challenges ahead: it may be necessary to drop unfit candidates. Hold frequent meetings to discuss plans and responsibilities. Nominate a medic, cook, mechanic, driver, navigator, etc. Ensure everyone is familiar with the equipment and that you carry spares.

RESEARCH

The more detailed your knowledge of the place and people, the better your chances. Study your maps carefully, gain as much knowledge of the terrain as possible: climate; weather conditions; river directions and speed of flow; how high are the mountains/hills; what kind of vege-tation/animal life can you expect?

PLANNING

Divide the project into phases: entry phase, objective and recovery. Clearly state the aim of each phase and work out a time scale. Plan for emergency procedures such as vehi-cle breakdown, illness and casualty evacuation.

Allow plenty of time when estimating the rate of progress. Pressure to keep to an over-ambitious schedule leads to exhaustion and errors of judgment.

The need to replenish water supplies from local sources will be a major factor in determining your route.

Make sure someone knows where you are planning to go and your times of departure and expected arrival. Keep them informed at prearranged stages so that failure to con-tact will set alarm bells ringing. Boats and aircraft are strictly controlled in this respect. If you are hiking in the hills inform the police and local mountain rescue center of your proposed plan.

Contingency plans

Be prepared in case anything goes wrong. What will you do if a vehicle breaks down, or if weather conditions prove more severe than anticipated? If in a party, how will you regroup if separated? What happens if someone falls ill?

EQUIPMENT

Clothes should be well-fitting but not restrictive, giving protection from cold and rain while keeping the body ven-tilated. Carry waterproofs, a change of clothes and extra warm garments. Layer in cold climates. Synthetics such as Gore-tex™ and fleece are versatile and useful. Wool is excellent in cold and wet climates, while cotton works well in the tropics.

Sleeping bag

Down bags are light and give better insulation than man-made fibers. When wet, however, down loses its insulating properties and is difficult to dry out. If you don't have a tent, a bivouac bag of "breathable" material will keep you dry.

Backpack

Must be strong, waterproof, with tough, adjustable webbing secured to the frame, and a comfortable belt to take the weight on the hips. External frames are best: although heavier and prone to snag on branches, they can take awkward, heavy loads, and even an injured person. The frame should allow an airspace between the pack and your back to reduce perspiration. Zip-fastened side pockets are best.

STOWING KIT

Pack so you know where everything is and the first things you need are on top. If it's wet, stow items in polythene bags. Tent and heavy kit go on top, but don't make the pack too high as it will be hard to balance in strong wind. Keep damageable food in containers.

RADIO

A necessity for long, remote expeditions. Prearrange a signals plan with twice-daily scheduled calls to base giving your location and plans. Base can supply weather updates and other info, and monitor the frequency for emergency calls if necessary. Select frequencies that will work in the areas you are going to. At least two group members should be able to operate the radio. An emergency plan will go into operation if you miss two consecutive calls from base. In this case, go to or stay at the last reported location and await contact.

G.P.S.

A G.P.S. (Global Positioning System) receives radio signals from satellites and can locate your current position anywhere in the world. They are relatively easy to use, and have a 95% accuracy rate. However, the satellite transmission must not have any obstructions in its way, so be sure to be standing still and out in the open when using your G.P.S. As with any battery-operated piece of equipment, do not use the G.P.S. as a substitute for basic navigation skills, but rather as a way of confirming or correcting your navigation.

MOBILES

Mobile phones offer a helpful supplement to radio contact, and can be a real life-saver in emergency situations. Check your network coverage before an expedition. Conserve batteries and protect from moisture. Remember, it takes less power to listen than to transmit.

SURVIVAL KIT

The items shown on p. 9 can make all the difference in the fight for survival. They should be stored in a small container, such as a 2 oz tobacco tin. Polish the inside of the lid to make a reflecting surface. Seal with a strip of adhesive tape (a) which can be easily removed and replaced to make it waterproof. Pack empty space with cotton wool (for fire lighting) to keep contents from rattling.

Check contents regularly, changing any which deteriorate. Never leave the tin open or lying on the ground. Make a habit of always having it with you.

1 **MATCHES** Preferably waterproof, but non-safety matches can be "shower proofed" by dipping heads in melted candle fat. Snap off half to save space.

2 **CANDLE** Shave square for packing. Tallow ones can be eaten in emergency or used for frying, but difficult to store in hot climates. Other kinds inedible.

3 **FLINT** Processed flint with saw striker.

4 **MAGNIFYING GLASS** To start fire in sunlight.

5 **NEEDLES AND THREAD** Several needles, including at least one with a very large eye to take sinew and coarse threads. Wrap length of strong thread around the needles.

6 **FISH HOOKS AND LINE** Selection of hooks and split lead weights, plus as much line as possible.

7 **COMPASS** Liquid-filled type with luminous button is best. Make sure it is in working order and that you know how to use it. Pointer is prone to rust: check it is on its pivot and swings freely.

8 **BETA LIGHT** A light-emitting crystal for map-reading at night and as fishing lure.

9 **SNARE WIRE** Preferably brass. 60–90 cm (2–3 ft).

10 **FLEXIBLE SAW** Remove handles and grease before storing. To use, fit wooden toggle handles.

11 **MEDICAL KIT** Pack medicines in airtight containers with cotton wool. Label carefully with full dosage instructions and expiration date. Do not exceed recommended dosages or take with alcohol. The following items are only a guide:

Analgesic Pain reliever for mild/moderate pain.

Intestinal sedative For acute/chronic diarrhea.

Antibiotic For general infections. Carry enough for a full course.

Antihistamine For allergies, insect bites/stings.

Water sterilizing tablets Use when you cannot boil suspect water.

Anti-malaria tablets Essential in areas where malaria is present.

Potassium permanganate Add to water and mix until pink to sterilize, deeper pink to make antiseptic, full red to treat fungal diseases, e.g., athlete's foot.

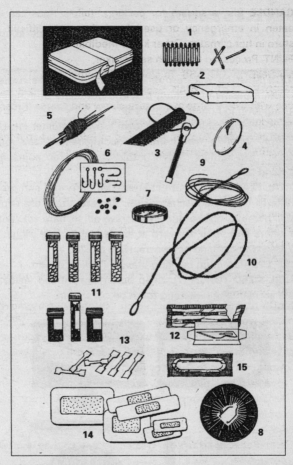

12 **SURGICAL BLADES** At least two scalpel blades of different sizes.

13 **BUTTERFLY SUTURES** To hold edges of wounds together.

14 **PLASTERS** Waterproof, assorted sizes.

15 **CONDOM** Makes good water-bag: holds 1 liter (2 pints).

SURVIVAL POUCH

In addition to your survival tin, pack a pouch and keep it handy for emergencies.

POUCH Must be waterproof, large enough to take a mess tin, with a positive fastening that will not come undone and a strong loop to hold it on your belt.

FUEL Solid fuel tablets in their own stove container (1). Use sparingly when a wood fire is inconvenient. They make excellent fire lighters. Stove unfolds to form an adjustable pot stand (2).

SIGNAL FLARES (3) to attract attention. Carry red and green miniflares (4) and a discharger (5). Beware: these are explosives! Remove discharger and screw on to flare (6). Withdraw flare and point skyward at arm's length. Pull trigger to fire. Use with care; do not waste. (See p. 220.)

MESS TIN Aluminum cooking utensil. Pack kit inside.

PENCIL-SIZED TORCH (7). Keep batteries reversed inside to avoid accidentally switching torch on.

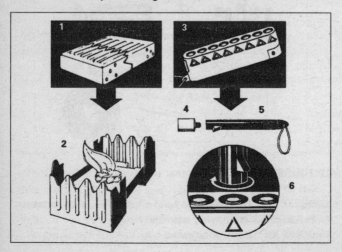

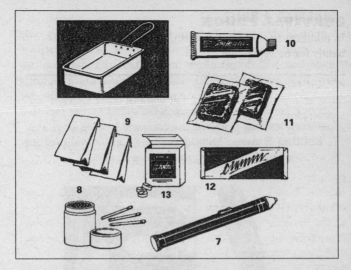

MARKER PANEL Fluorescent strip c. 0.3 x 2 m (1 x 6 ft) for signaling. (See p. 213.)

MATCHES (8) Pack in waterproof container.

BREW KIT Tea powder, sachets of milk and sugar (9).

FOOD Tube of butter (10). Dehydrated meat (11). Chocolate (12). Salt tablets (13) or electrolyte powder which contains vitamins, salt and other minerals.

SURVIVAL BAG Heat-insulated bag 200 x 60 cm (7 x 2 ft) of reflective material that keeps you warm and free of condensation.

SURVIVAL LOG Written log of all events. It will become a valuable reference and training tool.

KNIVES

A knife is an invaluable asset in a survival situation, but remember that knives are weapons and should be surrendered to airline staff when traveling by air. Never display in tense or awkward situations.

CHOOSING A KNIFE

A multi-bladed penknife is useful, but if you can carry only one knife take something stronger, a general-purpose blade that will do all likely tasks efficiently and comfortably, from cutting trees to skinning animals and preparing food. Some have built-in compasses or hollow handles for carrying kit, but any advantages are offset by the fact that such handles may break or the compass lose its accuracy.

Folding Knives: Should have a good locked position. A wooden handle is more comfortable to use.

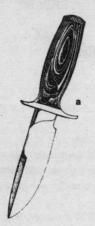

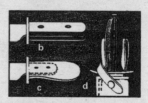

Handle (a) is ideal: a single rounded piece of wood, the knife tang passing through it and fastened at the end. Handle (b) is riveted and would cause blisters, (c) could easily break. The sheath (d) must have a positive fastening and tunnel belt loop.

You are only as sharp as your knife. It must be sharp and ready for use. Don't misuse your knife by throwing it. Keep it clean, oiled and in a sheath when not in use.

Parang: The Malayan name for a knife with a large curved blade like a machete. Too large for everyday use, it is ideal in the wilds for cutting down trees and building shelters and rafts. The ideal parang size is 30 cm (12 in) overall blade length, with a blade 5 cm (2 in) at its widest, weighing no more than 750 g (1.5 lb). The end of the blade should be bolted into a wooden handle.

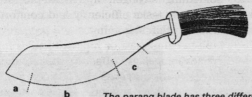

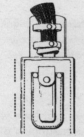

The parang blade has three different edges: (b) does the heavy work of chopping wood and bone; (a) is finer and used for skinning; (c) is for carving and delicate work. The curved blade enables maximum effort to be applied when cutting timber and the blade arrives before the knuckles, offering protection.

The sheath must have positive fastenings to keep the parang secure and a loop for fixing to a belt. Some sheaths have a pocket on the front for a sharpening stone.

 There is a danger that the cutting edge may come through the side of the sheath. NEVER hold the sheath on the same side as the cutting edge when drawing the parang. Always grip the side AWAY FROM THE CUTTING EDGE.

Sharpening a knife

Sandstone, quartz and granite will sharpen tools. Rub two pieces together to make them smooth. A double-faced stone with a rough and smooth surface is ideal. Use the rough surface first to remove burrs, then the smooth one to get a fine edge. The object is to get an edge that will last and not chip.

To sharpen the blade, hold the handle in the right hand. Use a clockwise circular motion and apply steady pressure on the blade with the fingertips of the left hand as you push away. Keep the angle constant and the stone wet. Don't drag the blade toward you under pressure; this produces burrs. Reduce the pressure for a finer edge. Work counterclockwise on the other side.

Blade profile: A is too steep and will soon wear; B is good; and C is too fine and will chip.

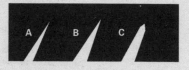

Get in the habit of checking all your equipment regularly, especially after negotiating difficult terrain. A check of all pockets and possessions should be second nature.

FACING DISASTER
It is no use giving up. Only positive action can save you. People can survive seemingly impossible situations if they have the determination.

SURVIVAL STRESSES
The survival situation will put you under physical and mental pressure. You will have to overcome some or all of the following stresses:

Fear and anxiety

Pain, illness and injury

Cold and/or heat

Thirst, hunger and fatigue

Sleep deprivation

Boredom

Loneliness and isolation

Can you cope? You have to.

Self-confidence is a product of good training and sound knowledge. These must be acquired before you face a survival situation. Confidence will help you overcome the mental stresses. Physical fitness will give you the resources to cope with fatigue and loss of sleep. The fitter you are the better you will survive. Start training now.

Pain and fever call attention to an injured part and prevent you using it. It is important to treat any injury as soon as possible, but pain may have to be overcome and controlled in order to seek help and avoid the risk of further injury or death.

WATER

Ordering your priorities is one of the first steps to survival. Our basic needs are food, fire, shelter and water. Their order of importance will depend on where you are, but water is always essential.

An adult can survive for three weeks without food but only three days without water. Don't wait until you run out of water before you look for more. Conserve supplies and seek a new source of fresh running water, though all water can be sterilized.

The human body loses 2–3 liters (4–6 pints) of water each day. Loss of liquids through respiration and perspiration increases with work rate and temperature. Vomiting and diarrhea increase loss further. This must be replaced either by actual water or water contained in food.

HOW TO RETAIN FLUIDS
To keep fluid loss to the minimum, take the following precautions:

Avoid exertion. Just rest. Don't smoke.

Keep cool. Stay in shade. If there is none, erect a cover to provide it.

Do not lie on hot ground or heated surfaces.

Don't eat, or eat as little as possible—digestion uses up fluids, increasing dehydration. Fat is especially hard to digest.

Never drink alcohol. This takes fluid from vital organs to break it down.

Don't talk. Breathe through the nose, not the mouth.

FINDING WATER

Look in valley bottoms where water naturally drains. If there is no stream or pool, look for patches of green vegetation and dig there.

Dig in gullies and dry stream beds.

In mountains look for water trapped in crevices.

On the coast dig above the high water line, or look for lush vegetation in faults in cliffs: you may find a spring.

 Be suspicious of any pool with no green vegetation growing around it, or animal bones present. It is likely to be polluted. Check edge for minerals which might indicate alkaline conditions. Always boil water from pools. In the desert, lakes with no outlets become salt lakes: their water must be distilled before drinking.

Dew and Rain Collection: Use as big a catchment area as possible, running the water off into containers. A covered hole in the ground lined with clay will hold water. If you have no impermeable sheeting, use metal sheets or bark to catch water.

Use clothing to soak up water: tie clean cloths around the legs and ankles and walk through wet vegetation. These can be sucked or wrung out.

RATION YOUR SWEAT, NOT YOUR WATER!
If you have to ration water, take it in sips. After going without water a long time, don't guzzle when you do find it. Take only sips at first. Large gulps will make a dehydrated person vomit, losing even more of the valuable liquid.

ANIMALS AS SIGNS OF WATER

Mammals

Most animals require water regularly. Grazing animals are usually never far from water as they need to drink at dawn and dusk. Converging game trails often lead to water; follow them downhill. Meat eaters are not good indicators—they get moisture from their prey.

Birds

Grain eaters, such as finches and pigeons, are never far from water and drink at dawn and dusk. When they fly straight and low they are heading for water. When returning from water they fly from tree to tree, resting frequently. Water birds and birds of prey do not drink frequently and are therefore not good indicators.

Insects

Bees are especially good indicators. They fly at most 6.5 km (4 miles) from their nests or hives. Ants are dependent on water. A column of ants marching up a tree is going to a small reservoir of trapped water. Such reservoirs are found even in arid areas. Most flies keep within 90 m (100 yards) of water.

Reptiles

They collect what little moisture they need from dew and their prey. Not good indicators.

Humans

Tracks usually lead to a well, bore hole or soak. It may be covered with scrub or rocks to reduce evaporation. Replace the cover.

CONDENSATION

Trees can draw moisture from a water table 15 m (50 ft) or more below ground, too deep for you to dig. Let the tree pump it up for you by tying a plastic bag around a healthy, leafy branch or placing a polythene tent over vegetation. Evaporation from the leaves will produce condensation in the bag.

Keep the mouth of the bag at the top with a corner hanging low to collect water.

Suspend tent from the apex or support with padded stick. Avoid foliage touching the sides or it will divert droplets from collecting in plastic-lined channels at the bottom.

Even cut vegetation will produce condensation when placed in a large plastic bag. Keep foliage off the bottom with stones so that water collects below it, and don't let it touch the sides. Keep the bag taut with stones. Support the top on a padded stick. Arrange the bag on a slight slope so condensation runs down to the collecting point.

Solar still

Dig a hole approximately 90 cm (36 in) across and 45 cm (18 in) deep. Place a collecting can in the center, then cover the hole with a sheet of plastic formed into a cone. Roughen underside of sheet with a stone to ensure droplets run down it. The sun raises the temperature of the air and soil below, producing vapor. Water condenses on the underside of the plastic, running down into the container. This is especially effective where it is hot by day and cold at night. This kind of still should collect at least 550 ml (1 pint) over a 24-hour period.

The still doubles as a trap. Insects and small snakes, attracted by the plastic, slide down into the cone or wriggle beneath it into the hole and cannot climb out.

A solar still can be used to distill pure water from poisonous or contaminated liquids.

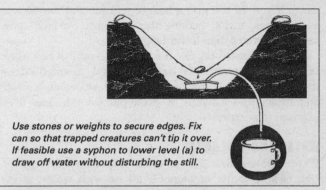

Use stones or weights to secure edges. Fix can so that trapped creatures can't tip it over. If feasible use a syphon to lower level (a) to draw off water without disturbing the still.

☠ URINE AND SEAWATER
Never drink either—never. But both can produce drinking water if distilled—and seawater will provide you with a residue of salt.

Distillation

Pass a tube into the top of a water-filled covered container, placed over a fire, and the other end into a sealed collecting tin which should be set inside another container providing a jacket of cold water to cool the vapor as it passes out of the tube. You can use any tubing, e.g., pack frames. To avoid wasting water vapor, seal around the joins with mud or wet sand.

An easier method is a variation on the desert still. Take a tube from a covered vessel in which polluted or salt water is to boil. Set the other end under a solar still. A sheet of metal, bark, or leaf weighted down, will cover the vessel and help direct the steam into the tube.

WATER FROM ICE AND SNOW

Ice produces twice as much water as snow for half the heat. To heat snow, melt a little in a pot and gradually add more. If you fill the pot, a hollow will form at the bottom as the snow melts, making the pot burn. Surface snow yields less water than lower layers.

Sea ice is salt—no use for drinking—until it has aged. Old sea ice is bluish and has weathered, rounded edges; the bluer it is the better for drinking. New sea ice is white and rough. But beware of even old ice that has been exposed to seaspray.

WATER FROM PLANTS

Water Collectors: Plants often trap water in cavities. Old, hollow joints of bamboo fill up with water: shake them—if you hear water, cut a notch at the base of each joint and tip the water out.

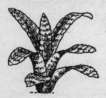

Cup-shaped plants catch and hold water, which should be strained to remove insects and debris.

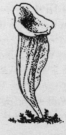

Bromeliads range from 5 cm–9 m (2 in–30 ft) high but most are 30–150 cm (1–5 ft). Some store water in their tissues and all collect it in a reservoir formed by leaf bases.

Vines: with rough bark and shoots about 5 cm (2 in) thick can be a useful source of water. But beware: not all have drinkable water and some yield a sticky, milky sap which is poisonous. Some vines cause skin irritation on contact, so collect the liquid in a container or let it drip into your mouth rather than put your mouth to the stem. To obtain water from a vine select a stem and trace it upward. Reach as high as possible and cut a deep notch in the stem. Cut off the same stem close to the ground and let the water drip from it. When it ceases to drip cut a section from the bottom and go on repeating this until the vine is drained. Do not cut the bottom of the vine first as this will cause the liquid to run up the vine through capillary action.

Roots: In Australia the water tree, desert oak and bloodwood have their roots near the surface. Pry the roots out and cut them up into 30 cm (12 in) lengths. Remove the bark. Suck out the moisture, or shave to a pulp and squeeze over the mouth.

Palms: The buri, coconut and nipa palms all contain a sugary fluid which is drinkable. To start it flowing bend a flowering stalk downward and cut off its tip. If a thin slice is cut off the stalk every 12 hours the flow will be renewed, making it possible to collect up to a quart each day. Nipa palms shoot from the base so that you can work from ground level, but on grown trees of other species you may have to climb up to reach a flowering stalk.

Coconut milk from ripe nuts is a powerful laxative; drinking too much would make you lose more fluid.

Cacti: Water is stored in the fruit and bodies, but some cacti are very poisonous. Avoid contact with the spines, which can be difficult to remove and can cause festering sores.

The barrel cactus can reach a height of 120 cm (4 ft) and is found in the southwestern United States through to

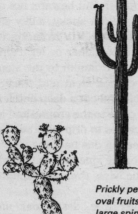

Saquarro cactus of Mexico and USA grows to 5 m (17 ft) and holds lots of poisonous liquid. Collect and place in a solar still to evaporate and recondense overnight.

Prickly pears have big "ears" and produce oval fruits which ripen to red or gold. Their large spines are easy to avoid. Both fruit and "ears" are moisture laden.

South America. The spine-covered outer skin is very tough: the best method is to cut off the top and chop out pieces from the inside to suck, or smash the pulp within the plant and scoop out the watery sap. A 100 cm (3.5 ft) barrel cactus will yield about 1 liter (2 pints) of milky juice and this is an exception to the rule to avoid milky-sapped plants.

WATER FROM ANIMALS

Animal eyes contain water which can be extracted by sucking them.

All fish contain a drinkable fluid. Large fish, in particular, have a reservoir of fresh water along the spine. Tap it by gutting the fish and, keeping the fish flat, remove the backbone, being careful not to spill the liquid, and then drink it.

If water is very scarce be careful not to suck up the other fish juices in the flesh, because they are rich in protein and fluid will be taken from your vital organs to digest them.

Desert animals can also be a source of moisture. In northwestern Australia, aborigines dig for desert frogs that burrow in the ground. They store water in their bodies and it can be squeezed out of them.

SALT

Salt is another essential for human survival. A normal diet includes a daily intake of 10 g (0.5 oz). The body loses salt in sweat and urine and you need to replace that loss.

> The first symptoms of salt deficiency are muscle cramps, dizziness, nausea and tiredness. The remedy is to take a pinch of salt in a pint of water. There are salt tablets in your survival kit. Break them up and dissolve in an appropriate amount in water. Do not swallow them whole as this can cause stomach upsets and kidney damage.

If your supplies run out and you are near the sea, salt water contains about 15 g (0.75 oz) of salt, but do not drink it as it is. Dilute it with plenty of fresh water to make it drinkable, or evaporate it to get salt crystals.

Inland, salt can be obtained from some plants such as the roots of hickory trees in North America or of the nipa palm in southeastern Asia. Boil the roots until all the water evaporates and black salt crystals are left.

If no direct salt sources are available then rely on getting it secondhand through animal blood, which is a valuable source of minerals.

SURVIVAL LOG

Keep a record of all events, particularly discoveries of edible plants and other resources. It becomes a valuable reference and making it helps keep up morale.

CLIMATE AND TERRAIN

T HIS chapter cannot provide a world geography, it can only summarize types of climate and terrain. It is vital to research conditions in areas you plan to visit, but a knowledge of climate zones will help if accident throws you into unfamiliar territory.

Temperate climates cover much of the globe, and offer the best chances for survival without special skills or knowledge. These territories are also the most heavily urbanized. Heavy winter conditions may call for polar skills.

CLIMATE ZONES

Polar regions: Technically, latitudes higher than 60°33′ north and south, but polar skills may be needed at very high altitudes everywhere. In addition to the poles, arctic conditions can occur in Alaska, Canada, Greenland, Iceland, Scandinavia, and the former USSR.

Tundra: Treeless zone south of the polar cap. The subsoil is permanently frozen and vegetation stunted.

Northern coniferous forest: Up to 1300 km (800 miles) deep, lies between arctic tundra and temperate lands. Winters are long and severe. Trees and plants flourish along the great rivers that flow to the Arctic Ocean. Game, ranging from elk and bear to squirrels and birds, is plentiful. Melted snow creates swamps in the brief summer. Fallen trees and dense growth make the going difficult, and mosquitoes can be a nuisance. Travel along rivers. Movement is easier in winter.

Deciduous forest: Oak, beech, maple and hickory are the main species in America; oak, beech, chestnut and lime, in Eurasia. The rich soil supports many plants. Survival is easy, except in very high altitudes where tundra or snowfield conditions apply.

Temperate grassland: Found in central continental areas of North America and Eurasia. Hot summers, cold winters and moderate rainfall have made these the great food-producing areas.

Mediterranean regions: Lands bordering the Mediterranean are semi-arid, with long hot summers and short dry winters. Trees are few, water is scarce.

Tropical forests: Equatorial rain forest, subtropical rain forest and montane forest all feature high rainfall and rugged mountains, which drain into large, swift-flowing rivers, with coastal and low-lying regions as swamp land.

Savannah: Tropical grassland found in Australia, Venezuela, Colombia, Brazil and Africa. Grass grows up to 3 m (10 ft). Temperatures are high all year round. Water is scarce, but where it is found there will be lush vegetation and plenty of wildlife.

Desert: One-fifth of the earth's land surface is desert, of which only small parts are sand; most is flat gravel cut by dried-up water courses (wadis). Very high temperatures occur by day, falling to below freezing at night. Survival is difficult.

POLAR REGIONS

Winter temperatures are well below freezing and hurricane-force winds can whip snow 30 m (100 ft) into the air. A 32 kmph (20 mph) wind brings a -14° C (5° F) thermometer

reading down to an actual temperature of -34° C (-30° F).
Days vary from total darkness mid-winter to 24-hour daylight midsummer.

TRAVEL

Establish shelter as near to the aircraft or vehicle as possible. Move only if rescue improbable. Cold dulls the mind—
plan while you can still think clearly.

Navigation is difficult in featureless terrain, and the
going treacherous. Don't move in a blizzard. Sea ice turns
to slush in summer and the tundra is boggy.

Don't make shelter near water, the habitat of black fly,
mosquito and deerfly. Cover skin, wear a net over the head
and burn green wood to keep them at bay.

Navigation

Compasses are unreliable near the Poles, so be guided
by the constellations and travel by night. By day use the
shadow stick method. (See p. 171.)

Do not use icebergs or distant landmarks to fix direction: floes move constantly, and relative positions change.
If breaking ice forces you to another floe, leap from and to
a spot at least 60 cm (2 ft) from the edge.

> Avoid icebergs—they can turn over without warning,
> particularly with your added weight. Avoid sailing close
> to ice-cliffs—huge masses of ice can break off without
> warning.

Observe birds: in the thaw wildfowl fly to land; seabirds
fly out to sea by day, returning at night.

Clouds over open water, timber or snow-free ground
appear black below; over sea ice and snowfields, white.
New ice produces grayish reflections, mottled ones indicate pack ice or drifted snow.

Follow rivers: travel downstream—by raft or on ice—except in N. Siberia where rivers flow north. On frozen rivers keep to edges and outer curve on bends. Where rivers join follow the outside edge or take to outer bank. If river has many bends, take to land.

> ☠ **ICE-COLD WATER IS A KILLER**
> **Falling into icy water knocks the breath out of you. The body loses muscular control, consciousness fades, death follows in 15-20 minutes. RESIST! Take action. Move fast for land. Roll in snow to absorb water. Get to shelter and dry kit at once.**

CLOTHING

Severe cold freezes exposed flesh in minutes. Cover every part of the body. Wear a drawstring hood; a fur trim prevents breath freezing on the face and injuring the skin. If clothing has no drawstrings, tie sleeves above cuffs, tuck trousers in to prevent heat escaping. If you sweat, loosen collar or cuffs, or remove a layer.

Outer garments should be windproof, but not waterproof, which could trap vapor inside—animal skins are ideal. Underlayers should trap air for insulation. Wool is best for inner garments. It does not absorb water and is warm even when damp. Cotton absorbs moisture and rapidly loses heat when wet.

Footwear

Mukluks, waterproof canvas boots with rubber soles, are ideal. They should have an insulated liner.

Wear 3 pairs of socks, graded in size to fit over each other and not wrinkle. To improvise footwear use layers of fabric. Canvas seat covers make good boots.

(See Trench foot, p. 263.)

Snow shoes: Skiing is fine for firm snow but snow

shoes are best in soft snow. Lift each foot without angling it, keeping shoe as flat to the ground as possible.

Bend a long green sapling back on itself to form a loop; secure ends firmly. Add cross-pieces and twine, but don't make the shoes too heavy. Allow a firmer central section to attach to your foot.

SHELTER

Get out of the wind! Look for natural shelter to improve on, but avoid sites where a snowdrift, avalanche or rock fall might bury you. Avoid snow-laden trees (branches may fall) unless lower boughs are supported (see p. 114).

Don't block every hole against draughts. You must have ventilation, especially if your shelter has a fire.

C.O.L.D.

The key to keeping WARM

Keep it   **C**lean—Dirt and grease block air spaces!

Avoid   **O**verheating—Ventilate!

Wear it   **L**oose—Allow air to circulate!

Keep it   **D**ry—Outside and inside!

FIRE

Fuel sources are limited: driftwood, seal and bird fat, fuel from wreckage—in extreme cold drain oil from sump before it congeals. Can be used solid if drained on ground. High octane fuel can be left in the tanks.

On the tundra, willow, birch scrub and juniper may be found. (See p. 122.)

Casiope is a low, spreading heather-like plant with tiny leaves and white bell-shaped flowers. It contains so much resin it burns when wet.

WATER

In summer water is plentiful. Pond water may look brown and taste brackish but vegetation growing in it keeps it fresh. If in doubt, boil it.

In winter melt ice and snow. Do not eat crushed ice, it can injure your mouth and cause further dehydration. Thaw snow enough to mold into a ball before sucking it.

Remember—if you are already cold and tired, eating snow will further chill your body.

FOOD

Best chances for survival are along coasts where food supplies—fish, seals, seabirds—are dependable.

Antarctic: Lichens and mosses are the only plants. Most birds migrate in autumn, but penguins stay. They are easiest to catch when nesting.

Arctic: Arctic foxes sometimes follow polar bears to scavenge their kills. Northern wildlife is migratory and availability depends on season.

Tundra and Forest: Plants and animals available year round. Tundra plants are small compared to temperate species.

> **POISONOUS PLANTS**
> The majority of Arctic plants are edible but avoid water hemlock, baneberry and arctic buttercups. Other poisonous species include lupin, monkshood, larkspur, vetch, false hellebore and death camas. Best avoid fungi too—make sure you can distinguish lichens from them!

ANIMALS FOR FOOD

Caribou (reindeer), musk-ox and elk (moose) inhabit the Arctic, as do wolves, beaver, mink, wolverines and weasels. Foxes, living in the tundra in summer and open woodland in winter, are an indication of other, smaller prey—mountain hares, squirrels and small burrowing rodents.

Bears and walruses are very dangerous. Leave them alone unless you are armed.

Hunting and trapping

Tracks in snow are easy to follow, but leave a trail of bright flags to guide you back to base. Make them high enough not to be covered by a fresh snowfall.

Caribou can be lured by waving a cloth and moving on all fours. Ground squirrels and marmots may run to you if you are between them and their holds. Kissing the back of your hand makes a sound like a wounded mouse or bird and attracts prey. Find a concealed, downwind position. Be patient. Keep trying.

If you have a projectile weapon (gun, bow, catapult) which can be fired from ground level, lie in ambush behind a screen of snow, or make a screen of cloth.

Owls, ravens and ptarmigans are relatively tame and easy prey in winter. Many birds have a summer molt which makes them flightless. Eggs are edible at any stage of embryo development.

Seals provide food, clothing, and blubber. They are most vulnerable on the ice with their pups (produced March–June). Newborn pups cannot swim. Out of the breeding season, catch seals by their cone-shaped breathing holes (narrower on the upper surface of the ice). In thick ice flipper and toothmarks show where the seal has been keeping the hole open. Club the animal, then enlarge the hole to recover the carcass.

Polar bears feed on seals and fish. Most are curious and will come to you. Treat with respect and caution.

Always cook meat: muscles carry Trichinosis worm. Never eat seal or polar bear liver, which can have lethal concentrations of vitamin A.

PREPARING MEAT

Bleed, gut and skin while carcass is warm. Roll hides before they freeze. Cut meat into usable portions and freeze. Do not reheat meat—eat leftovers cold. Leave fat on all animals except seals. Remove seal fat; render it down before it can turn rancid and spoil meat.

Rodents—squirrels, rabbits—carry Tularemia, which can be caught from ticks or handling infected animals. Wear gloves when skinning. Boil meat.

ARCTIC HEALTH

Frostbite, hypothermia and snow blindness are the main hazards. Efforts to exclude drafts in shelters can lead to lack of oxygen and carbon monoxide poisoning.

Thinking can become sluggish. Keep alert and active, but avoid fatigue and conserve energy for useful tasks. Sleep as much as possible—you won't freeze in your sleep unless you are so exhausted you cannot regenerate the heat you lose to the air. Exercise fingers and toes to improve circulation. Take precautions against frostbite (see p. 262).

Avoid spilling petrol on bare flesh; it will freeze at once and damage the skin.

Don't put off defecation—this can cause constipation. Try to time it conveniently before leaving your shelter so you can take waste out with you.

Snow glare can cause blindness. Protect the eyes with goggles or a strip of cloth or bark with narrow slits cut for eyes. Blacken underneath the eye with charcoal to reduce glare further.

MOUNTAINS

Snow-covered peaks offer no food or shelter. Climbing and negotiating icefields call for skills which must be learned in mountaineering schools.

If disaster strands you on a mountainside and rescue is unlikely, travel by day to the valleys where food and shelter are available. At night and in bad visibility this is too dangerous. Find shelter until visibility improves.

Shelter among rocks or wreckage (see p. 103). Salvage blankets from a crashed plane and cover up to prevent exposure. A plastic bag makes an improvised sleeping bag. On stony ground sleep on your stomach; on a slope sleep with your head uphill.

JUDGING TERRAIN

As you descend it is difficult to see what is below. Try moving along a spur to see what is below. The far side of a valley will give you an idea of what's on your side. The ground can fall steeply between a distant slope and a foreground bluff. Scree slopes are deceptive, appearing continuous until you are very close to a cliff.

DESCENT

Negotiating cliffs without a rope is very dangerous. Never attempt a high cliff. In the event of a plane crash it is less risky to wait for rescue than to climb.

On steep cliffs face the rock. For less steep rock faces with deep ledges, adopt a sideways position using the inside of your hand for support. For easier crags, descend facing outward with the body bent and where possible carry weight on the palms of the hands.

Descending by rope

With a rope it is possible to rappel down sheer cliffs. Use a doubled rope unless someone is left above to untie it or you are prepared to leave it behind, in which case use an undoubled rope for twice the descent.

Abseiling: Loop rope around a firm anchor (test with full body weight). Avoid sharp edges. Pass both ends of rope between legs from front, bring around to left of body, over right shoulder and down across back. Hold rope in front with left hand and at back with right. Plant feet firmly against slope about 45 cm (18 in) apart, and lean back. Let rope around body carry your weight. Do not try to support yourself with your upper hand. Step slowly downward. The lower hand controls rate of descent. Pay the rope out one hand at a time.

Make sure you are in a firm position before hauling the rope down and that you have planned your next move. Once the rope is down you may have no way of retracing your steps.

Abseiling can be dangerous. If possible, pad out shoulders and groin, and use gloves to prevent damage from friction. Never attempt unless accompanied by an expert or in a survival situation.

ASCENT

Climbing up, holds are easier to see, but it is safer to go around than over obstacles to avoid getting stuck. Plot a route from the bottom; keep body away from the rock, feet flat, and look up. Don't overstretch. Always keep three points of contact. Reach for a hold with one hand or foot, test it and seek a hold for the next hand.

To ascend fissures use the chimney technique. Place your back against one surface and wedge your legs across the gap to the other. Slowly move up.

Ascending with ropes
Belaying: One person makes the ascent with a light line

attached around the waist with a bowline, then hauls up the rope. At each stage of the ascent there must be a ledge to accommodate everyone and a tree or rock for an anchor. Secure the rope with a loop tied in a figure-of-eight or an overhand knot.

Belayer ties on with a bight (loop) or two bights to steady himself, and passes climbing rope over head and down to hips, making a twist around the arm closest to the anchor and takes up any slack. Climber ties on with a bowline around waist and begins to mount. Belayer takes in rope to keep it taut. Anchor, belayer and climber should be in a straight line.

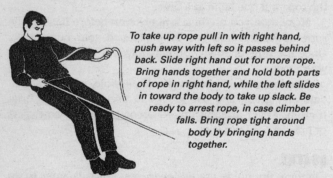

To take up rope pull in with right hand, push away with left so it passes behind back. Slide right hand out for more rope. Bring hands together and hold both parts of rope in right hand, while the left slides in toward the body to take up slack. Be ready to arrest rope, in case climber falls. Bring rope tight around body by bringing hands together.

FALLING ROCK CAN KILL
On loose rock always test holds gently and never pull outward on a loose hold. Be careful that your rope does not dislodge rocks. Even small falling rocks can inflict serious injury. If you knock a piece down, shout a warning to those below.

SNOW AND ICEFIELDS

If not equipped with proper ice axe and crampons and skilled in their use, try to keep clear of mountain ice.

On steep slopes climb in zigzags, kicking steps and drive snow axe or stick in sideways for stability. For gentle slopes dig in heels and use walking stick. On steep slopes descend backward driving stick into snow for support and as a brake if you slip. Never use this method where there is any risk of avalanche.

Security ropes: A party crossing a glacier should be tied together at not less than 9 m (30 ft) intervals. The leader should probe the snow with a stick for crevasses. Ropes fixed to a firm anchor at both ends can prevent falls: tie short rope around waist in a bowline and tie on to main rope with a prusik knot. This will slide along to allow descent but will arrest any falls.

If one of the group falls into a crevasse he must be hauled out with care: pressure of a rope on the chest can cause asphyxiation. Pass a looped rope down to put a foot in to take the weight. If the faller is unconscious three people in manharness hitches will be needed to pull him out. Speed is vital: temperatures in a crevasse are very low and the victim will rapidly weaken.

AVALANCHES

Avalanches are a serious hazard in all high mountain regions. They usually occur on slopes of 30°–45° within 24 hours of a snowfall. After a major fall of several hours' duration, wait a day for snow to settle. Rain or a rise in temperature after a snowfall increases the risk, as does heavy snow falling in low temperatures, because it does not have time to stabilize.

MAIN AREAS OF DANGER
Snow-covered convex slopes.
Lee slopes where snow has accumulated.
Deep snow-filled gullies.

PRECAUTIONS

Irregular, or timbered slopes are safest.

The heat of the sun on snow can cause avalanches, so before noon travel in shaded areas, while after noon, keep to slopes that have already been exposed to sun.

Avoid small gullies and valleys with steep side walls.

Stick to ridges and high ground above avalanche paths—you are more likely to trigger a slide but, if you do, have a better chance of being on top of the debris or not being carried down at all.

When crossing dangerous ground, rope together and use belays, always keeping at least 50 feet apart.

Always look out for avalanche activity, even if you do not see it happening. Assess where avalanches started, their direction, and how long ago they took place. They will be a guide to where other avalanches are likely to occur.

SEASHORES

Most seashores offer abundant sources of food and excellent prospects for survival.

Sandy beaches: Burrowing species—mollusks, crabs, worms—are left below the sand when the water recedes. They attract feeding birds.

It may be possible to find fresh water in the dunes and it is here that plants will grow. Dunes tend to be full of insects, so don't make camp there.

Muddy shores and estuaries: Where a river joins the sea it deposits sediment, forming large mud flats. These support many species of worms and mollusks and provide a feeding ground for birds and animals.

Rocky shores: If the cliffs are not too sheer, rock-pools may form—these teem with life. Rocks form an anchor for weed and sea urchins and crevices where octopus and other cephalopods can live.

Soft rocks, such as chalk, marl and limestone, erode quickly and have smooth surfaces. Hard rocks fracture in chunks and provide good nesting sites for birds.

Pebble beaches: Continual movement of pebbles makes a difficult habitat for most plants and animals.

Tides vary according to location and season.

HIGH-TIDE LEVEL INDICATORS

A line of debris along the beach.

Change in sand texture.

Weed, shells and color changes on cliff faces.

SHORE SAFETY

Time the tides and study their pattern to avoid being cut off by an incoming tide or swept out by the ebb.

Always check access from a beach or rocky shore. Keep an eye on the tide so you do not get cut off.

Look out for strong currents, especially off headlands. Sandbanks and submerged rocks are also dangerous. Where a beach falls steeply into deep water there will be a strong undertow. If you enter the water, have a safety line around the waist and a firm anchor on shore.

SWIMMING

When fishing or swimming stay within your depth and watch for large waves which can knock you off your feet. If caught in the undertow of a large wave, push off the bottom and swim to the surface. Swim to shore in the trough between waves. When the next wave comes, face it and submerge. Let it pass and swim in the next trough shoreward.

If forced off shore by a strong current do not fight it—swim across it, using side stroke, and make for land farther along the coast. Side stroke is not the strongest or fastest stroke, but it is the least tiring.

If being swept on to rocks, face land, adopt sitting position, feet first to absorb the shock. Wear shoes.

> A relaxed body floats best, so stay calm. It is difficult to sink in saltwater. The main danger is in swallowing the water. Women are more buoyant than men and float naturally on their backs. Men float naturally face down, but don't forget to lift your head out to breathe!

WATER

Fresh water is best obtained from small river outlets—large rivers tend to be polluted and full of silt.

Seek pools among dunes (see p. 16).

Freshwater rock pools can be identified by the growth of green algae which is not grazed by mollusks (saltwater mollusks cannot survive in fresh water).

Look for water trickling through rock, especially where mosses and ferns grow—it will be drinkable.

If stranded on a rocky outcrop offshore the only source of water may be the sea. Never drink seawater without distilling it. It can be used for cooking—but do not eat until you have a supply of fresh water.

FOOD

Hunt for fish and mollusks in rock pools at low tide, and dig for mollusks and other creatures in sand.

Only eat mollusks collected live. Bivalves (oysters, mussels, etc.) should close tightly if tapped. Gastropods, (winkles, whelks) have a trap-door entrance to the shell, which should close tightly if the shell is shaken. Limpets and abalones are anchored to rocks. Pry off with a knife. If they are hard to dislodge they are good to eat—only sick or dead ones come off easily.

> Bivalves can build up dangerous concentrations of toxic chemicals in polluted areas. In tropical zones mussels are poisonous in summer, especially when seas are reddish or phosphorescent. In the Arctic, black mussels are poisonous at any time of year.

Don't expose yourself to parasites and pollutants: cook shell foods by boiling for at least five minutes.

On most coasts the best time to fish from the shore is about two hours after high water. Make use of the tide by building fish traps (see p. 97).

Hunt octopus at night: attract them with a light, then spear them. To kill an octopus, turn it inside out: place hand inside the fleshy hood, grab the innards and pull hard—alternatively, stab it between the eyes, or bang it against a rock. The flesh is tough but nourishing. Boil the body and roast the tentacles.

Seashore plants differ according to the climate. Gather when weather or tide prevent you taking food from the sea.

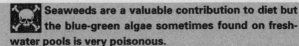 Seaweeds are a valuable contribution to diet but the blue-green algae sometimes found on freshwater pools is very poisonous.

Sea cucumbers live on the seabed or in the sand. They look like warty black cucumbers, up to 20 cm (8 in) long. Boil for five minutes. Sea urchins cling to rocks just below the low-water mark. Boil, split open and eat the egg-like inside, but avoid if their spines don't move when touched or if they smell bad when opened.

You can also fish for seabirds by leaving baited hooks among offal on flat rocks or throwing baited hooks into the air to be taken on the wing. Hunt on the ground for eggs that are easy to collect before risking raiding cliff nests.

See also *Reptiles* and *Crustaceans* (p. 64 and p. 102).

DANGERS

Beware in water too murky to see through. Wear shoes when foraging to protect from spines, which can inflict a painful wound. If you get pricked and the spine breaks off, trying to squeeze it out may push it in deeper. Most will work their way out after a few days.

Well-camouflaged creatures like stingrays can lie hidden: prod the bottom with a stick and stir up sand and rocks in front of you as you go. Stingray wounds can be soothed with very hot water.

Don't put your hands into underwater crevices—you could get bitten.

Always approach a coral reef with caution. Both the reef and its inhabitants—e.g., cone shells, which shoot a poisonous barb—can present dangers.

Lagoon fish are often poisonous—even species which are edible in the open sea. Fish from the reef on the seaward side of the lagoon instead.

If stung by a jellyfish do not pull the tentacles off or wipe away the slime with your hand—you will only get stung more. Use seaweed or a cloth, or wipe the sting with sand.

Octopuses have a hard beak and a few can give a poisonous bite, e.g., the blue-ringed octopus.

Shark attacks occur in very shallow water. Beware!

Keep clear of snakes in the water—they are highly poisonous. If found on shore, pin them with a forked stick—they make a good meal.

ISLANDS

Islands offer a special challenge, with acute isolation to be overcome. Explore the island and establish a daily routine. If it has been inhabited in the past, remains of buildings will offer shelter. If you find caves make sure they are not tidal and won't be flooded or cut off by spring tides, which are higher than normal.

On a barren outcrop shelter may simply mean finding a place out of the wind. Food will be whatever clings to the rocks and what you can haul from the sea.

RESOURCES

Take care not to over-exploit limited resources. Lack of water is the reason many islands are uninhabited. Catch and store rainwater and distill seawater. Lush vegetation is a sign of springs and streams.

Distilling seawater takes lots of fuel, e.g., driftwood, dried seaweeds, or seal blubber. Have a fire only when necessary. Search beaches after every tide for flotsam.

Coconut palms

Tropical islands are rarely desert islands—they usually offer plenty to eat. Coconut palms grow throughout the tropics and subtropics, providing fronds for shelter, husks for ropes, and milk and meat.

To remove the husk, force it over a sharpened stake or split it with a hand axe. Extract the milk by piercing one of the dark eyes of the nut before smashing it open to get at the meat. Coconut milk is safe and refreshing—a large nut may hold 1 liter (2 pints). Do not drink from young (green) or old (dark brown) nuts as there is a risk of diarrhea. The meat is indigestible in large amounts: eat a little at a time. Extract the oil by exposing chopped white meat to heat—sun or fire—and collecting oil as it runs off, or by boiling and skimming the oil as it rises to the surface. Rub it on to protect against sunburn and chafing from saltwater, to repel insects, as a salve for sores and blisters or, mixed with wood ash, as soap.

Climbing palms: If you need to climb to reach nuts, tie a strap of strong cloth and slip it around your ankles. Adjust it to hold your feet close to the trunk and press the soles of your feet inward to grip the tree.

ATTRACTING RESCUE

Lay out signals by arranging rocks, seaweed or anything that contrasts with surroundings.

Polish metal with sand to make signaling mirrors.

If you see a ship, try to make contact on a VHF radio.

MOVING ON

In a group of islands, you may be able to move on when resources are exhausted on the first. If land is in sight, study tides and currents. Float something you can observe and note its progress. It may be possible to swim, but use a flotation aid, e.g., an empty box or coconuts. Time your swim so the ebb takes you out from your island and the high tide takes you to the new island. Build a raft in cold climates—from autumn to spring seal carcasses will float; lash several together to support your weight.

ARID REGIONS

To survive you must make the most of any available shade, create protection from the sun, cut moisture loss and restrict activity during the heat of the day.

Where great temperature differences between night and day occur, condensation is a source of water.

When rain does come—years can pass with none at all—it may be in torrential downpours which create flash floods, before being quickly absorbed.

Dust or sandstorms reduce visibility. Protection is needed against sand entering every orifice.

WATER

Water is vital. If you have it, ration it immediately. If you are stranded by mechanical failure during a desert crossing, you will have planned your route with an awareness of oases, wells and waterholes. Wells may require a container lowered on a line to reach water. Small waterholes in wadi (watercourse) bottoms are often seasonal. They are usually covered with a stone or brushwood.

Away from known waterholes, dig at the lowest point of the outside bend of a dry streambed or the lowest point between dunes. Do not dig in the heat of day—you'll sweat liquid you may not be able to replace. Always balance fluid loss against possible gain. (See p. 15.)

Life expectancy depends on the water available and your ability to minimize perspiration. Without water you will last 2 days at 48° C (120° F) if you rest in the shade and do nothing. If you must walk to safety the distance you cover will relate to the water available. With none, a temperature of 48° C, walking at night and resting by day, you could cover 40 km (25 miles). Walking by day you would cover 8 km (5 miles) before collapse. At 48° C with 2 liters (4 pints) of water you might cover 56 km (35 miles) and last 3 days.

Drink 1.5 liters for every 2 lost (3:4 pints). Less fluid will not result in less sweat. If more fluid is drunk than needed it will be excreted and used to no purpose.

SHELTER AND FIRE

Find immediate shade. In the evening cool build a shelter. Do not stay in a metal vehicle or plane. Use it to support a shelter or make use of the shadow beneath an aircraft's wing. Pile rocks to make a windbreak and make use of wadi walls (except when flash floods seem likely). Use the double-layer technique to aid cooling (see p. 107). If using fabrics, leave bottom edges lifted and loose by day to increase air circulation. Weight them down with rocks at night. Avoid lying directly on hot ground: air can circulate under a raised bed.

You will need fire for warmth at night and for boiling water. Smoke will be useful for signaling. Desert scrub is dry and burns easily. If the land is totally barren, vehicle fuel and oil mixed with sand in a container will burn. Animal dung is also flammable.

CLOTHING

Clothing helps reduce fluid loss and gives protection from sunburn and insect bites, as well as warmth at night. Clothes should be light and loose fitting, with air space between the garments and the body. Copy the flowing, layered garments of the Arab world. Trousers give more protection from insects and guard against serious sunburn on the legs. Cover the head and feet.

> **Keep covered! Apart from risking severe sunburn, an uncovered body will lose sweat by evaporation. Keep clothing loose with a layer of insulating air. Sweating will then cool you more efficiently.**

Headgear: A hat with a piece of cloth attached to the back will protect but, better still, copy Arab headwear: make a handkerchief into a wad on top of the head, fold diagonally a piece of cloth about 120 cm (4 ft) square, place it over the handkerchief, long edge forward, and secure with a cord tied around head. This traps pockets of air, and protects from sand. Wrap around the face for warmth at night.

Eye protection: Sunglasses may not be enough. Soot from the fire smeared below the eyes will reduce glare. Shield eyes from glare and windborne sand with a strip of material. Cut narrow slits to see through.

Footwear: Do not walk barefoot until your feet have hardened or they will burn and blister. Do not leave tops of feet exposed. Puttees keep sand out of boots; wrap them around the feet over open sandals.

FOOD

Heat causes loss of appetite—don't force yourself to eat. Protein foods increase metabolic heat and water loss. If water is scarce, keep eating to a minimum and try to eat only moisture-containing foods, e.g., fruit and vegetables. Food spoils quickly in the desert. Once open, eat stores at once or keep covered and shaded.

Vegetation is scarce, but deserts often support a variety of animal life. Insects, reptiles, rodents and some small mammals burrow or hide during the day. Large mammals are an indication that there is water close at hand.

HEALTH

Most desert illnesses are caused by excessive exposure to sun and heat. They can be avoided by keeping head and body covered and remaining in the shade.

Constipation and pain in passing urine are common and salt deficiency can lead to cramps.

Heavy sweating coupled with garments that rub can block the sweat glands and result in an uncomfortable skin irritation known as prickly heat.

Heat cramps, leading to heat exhaustion, heat stroke and serious sunburn are all dangers. A gradual increase in activity and daily exposure to the sun will build up a defense, provided that plenty of drinking water is available.

Keep moist areas of the body—crevices of armpits, groin and toes—clean and dry to prevent infection.

☠ DESERT SORES

Even the most trivial wound will become infected if not dealt with straight away. Pull out thorns as soon as possible. Where the skin is broken a large and painful sore may develop which could prevent walking. Bandage all cuts with clean dressings and use what medical aids are available.

TROPICAL REGIONS

Everything in the jungle thrives, including disease and parasites. Even if saturated by perspiration, clothing affords protection from stings and bites.

Except at high altitudes, equatorial and subtropical regions are characterized by high temperatures, heavy rainfall and oppressive humidity. Violent storms may occur toward the end of the summer. In choosing camp sites make sure you are above potential flooding.

Equatorial rain forests: Temperatures range from 30° C (86° F) to 20° C (68° F) at night. Jungle trees rise from buttress roots to 60 m (200 ft). In this primary jungle the canopy prevents light reaching the jungle floor. It is relatively cool, with little undergrowth to hamper movement, but visibility is limited. It is easy to lose a sense of direction and difficult for rescuers to spot you.

Secondary jungle: Along riverbanks and the fringes of the jungle sunlight does penetrate to the floor and growth is prolific. Undergrowth reaches heights of 3 m (10 ft) in a year. Moving is slow, hot work, hacking a way with a parang or machete (see p. 188).

Subtropical rain forests: Found within 10° of the Equator, these forests have a season of reduced rainfall, even drought, with monsoons coming in cycles. More deciduous trees grow here and undergrowth is dense.

Rescue signals must be set in clearings (often found near river bends), or—better—on rafts on the river.

Montane forests: At altitudes above 1000 m (3000 ft). The Ruwenzori Range of central Africa is typical: a crater-like landscape covered in moss between ice-capped peaks. Plant growth is sparse, trees stunted and distorted. Low branches make the going hard. Nights are cold, days hot and misty. Survival is difficult: make your way down the slopes to tropical rain forest.

Saltwater swamps: In coastal areas subject to tidal flooding, mangrove trees thrive, reaching heights of 12 m (40 ft). Their tangled roots are an obstacle above and below the waterline. Visibility is low and passage difficult. Sometimes channels are wide enough to raft, but generally progress is on foot. You won't starve—fish, mollusks, aquatic animals and vegetation are plentiful—but it is a hostile environment with water leeches, cayman and crocodiles. Where river channels intersect the swamp you may be able to make a raft.

If forced to stay in a swamp determine the high-tide

level by the line of salt and debris on the trees, and fit a raised bed above it. Cover yourself for protection against ants and mosquitoes. Build your fire on a platform using standing deadwood for fuel. Decay is rapid in a swamp—choose wood that is not rotten.

Freshwater swamps: Found in low-lying inland areas, their thorny undergrowth makes the going difficult and reduces visibility—but survival is easy and swamps are often dotted with islands so you won't be chest deep in water all the time. There are often navigable channels and raw materials available from which to build a raft.

SHELTER
There are ample materials for building shelter in most tropical regions. Where temperatures are high and shelters exposed to the sun, make roofs in two layers with an airspace 20–30 cm (8–12 in) between to aid cooling. Double layers of cloth will help keep out rain if angled (see p. 107).

FIRE
Everything is likely to be damp. Take standing dead wood, shave off the outside and use that to start your fire. Dry bamboo and termite nests make good tinder.

FOOD
A wide variety of fruits, roots and leaves are available. Banana, papaya, mango and figs are easily recognized, but you may find the wealth of tropical foods bewildering. If you're not sure, use the tests described on p. 53 before you risk eating plants.

A wide range of mammals, reptiles, birds and fish can be hunted, trapped and fished (see pp. 56–102). Fish are easily digested, but in the tropics they spoil quickly. Clean thoroughly, discard entrails and eat as soon as possible. Do not preserve them by smoking or drying.

Fish in slow-moving water may be infested with tape-worms and other human parasites: boil for 20 minutes. Water itself may be infected with amoebas which cause dysentery: always boil.

DANGERS

INSECT ATTACK

Slashing your way through the jungle you may disturb bee, wasp or hornet nests. Any bare skin is vulnerable to attack. Run! Don't drop anything—you won't want to go back for it. Goggles will protect the eyes.

Insects, desperate for salt, will make for the sweaty parts of your body. Protect armpits and groin against their painful stings.

MOSQUITO PROTECTION

Wear a net or T-shirt over your head, especially at dawn and dusk. Better, take a strip of cloth 45 cm (18 in) deep and long enough to tie around your head; cut it to make a fringe of vertical strips hanging from a band that will dangle around your face and over your neck.

Keep covered at night, including your hands. Oil, fat or mud spread on hands and face may help repel insects.

Use bamboo or a sapling to support a tent of clothing and large leaves rigged over your upper half.

A smoky fire will help keep insects at bay.

COVER YOUR FEET

Good footwear and protection for the legs is essential. Wrap bark or cloth around legs and tie it to make put-tees as a defense against leeches and centipedes.

BEWARE HAIRY CATERPILLARS

Always brush off in the direction they are traveling or small irritant hairs may stay in your skin and cause an itchy rash, which may fester in the heat.

BEWARE INVADERS

Keep clothing and footwear off the ground so that scorpions, snakes and spiders don't creep in. Shake out clothes and check boots before putting them on; be wary when putting hands in pockets. Take care on waking: centipedes nestle for warmth in the more private body regions. Protect armpits and groin against stinging insects attracted by sweat.

LEECHES

Their bite is messy but not painful. Left alone they drop off when they have had their fill. Do not pull them off—the head may come off leaving the jaws in the bite, which could turn septic. Remove with a dab of salt, alcohol or a burning cigarette end, ember or flame.

BEWARE THE CANDIRU

This minute, almost transparent Amazonian catfish, about 2.5 cm (1 in) long, are reported to be able to swim up the urethra of a person urinating in the water—where it gets stuck by its dorsal spine. The chance of this happening is remote, but don't take the risk. Cover your genitals and don't urinate in the water.

RIVER DANGERS

Rivers can be home to dangerous creatures such as piranhas, stingrays and electric eels. Look out for crocodiles or alligators and take care in handling catfish, which have sharp dorsal fins and spines on their gill covers.

See p. 254 for first aid procedures if bitten or stung.

FOOD

THE survivor must understand the body's nutritional needs and how to meet them. This chapter provides details of how to trap, snare, hunt and fish, along with a miniature field guide to edible plants.

FOOD VALUES

A healthy body can survive on reserves stored in its tissues, but food is needed to supply heat and energy, and to recover after hard work, injury or sickness. Seventy calories per hour are required just for breathing and basic bodily functions. Work or major activity can burn up over 5,500 calories daily. Save calories: do not squander energy.

> A balanced diet is as important as having enough to eat. Vary your diet: it must include a range of elements which provide the right proportions of fat, protein, carbohydrates, minerals and vitamins.

Carbohydrates: Easily digested, a primary source of energy, they prevent ketosis (nausea due to breakdown of body fats). They come in two forms: sugars, found in sugar, syrup, honey, treacle and fruits; and starches, roots, tubers (always cook) and cereals. One gram (0.035 oz) produces 4 calories.

Fats: A concentrated form of energy. Lengthy digestive process requires plenty of water. Found in animals, fish, eggs, milk, nuts and some vegetables and fungi. One gram (0.035 oz) produces 9 calories.

Proteins: Main sources are meat, fish, eggs, dairy produce, nuts, grains, pulses and fungi. One gram (0.035 oz) produces 4 calories

Minerals: Phosphorus, calcium, sodium, potassium, chlorine, magnesium and sulphur are among those required in quantity. Only small amounts are needed of fluorine, iron and iodine. All are vital to good health.

Trace elements: These include strontium, aluminum, arsenic, gold and tiny amounts of other chemicals.

Vitamins: About a dozen are essential for humans. Vitamins D and K are synthesized by the body, but most come from external sources. Scurvy, beri-beri, rickets and pellagra all result from vitamin deficiency. Vitamin A aids vision and prevents eye disease.

FOOD PLANTS

There are few places without some kind of vegetation which can be eaten. Plants contain vitamins, minerals, protein and carbohydrates. Some contain fat and all provide roughage.

> Do not assume that because birds or mammals have eaten a plant it is edible by humans. Monkeys give some indication but no guarantee that plants are safe.

TESTING NEW PLANTS

Always adopt the following procedure when trying new plants as food. Never take shortcuts. One person only should complete the whole test. If in any doubt at any stage of the test, do not eat.

EDIBILITY TEST

INSPECT: Try to identify. Ensure the plant is not slimy or worm-eaten. Don't risk old, withered plants.

SMELL: Crush a small portion. If it smells of bitter almonds or peaches—discard it.

SKIN IRRITATION: Squeeze some juice or rub slightly on tender skin (e.g., under upper arm). If discomfort, rash or swelling is experienced, discard it.

LIPS, MOUTH, TONGUE: If there is no irritation so far, proceed to the following stages, waiting 15 seconds between each to check that there is no reaction:

- Place a small portion on lips
- Place a small portion in corner of mouth
- Place a small portion on tip of tongue
- Place a small portion under tongue
- Chew a small portion

In all cases, if discomfort is felt, e.g., soreness to throat, irritation, stinging or burning, discard it.

SWALLOW: Ingest a small amount and wait five hours. During this time drink or eat nothing else.

EATING: If no reactions, e.g., soreness to mouth, repeated belching, nausea, stomach or abdominal pains are experienced, plant may be considered safe.

Should stomach trouble occur, drink plenty of hot water; do not eat again until the pain goes. If it is severe, induce vomiting by tickling the back of the throat. Swallowing some charcoal will also induce vomiting and may absorb the poison at the same time. White wood ash mixed to a paste with water will relieve stomach pain.

GATHERING PLANTS

Gather plants systematically. Take a container on foraging trips to stop the harvest being crushed, which makes it go off.

Leaves and stems: Young growth will be tastier and more tender. Old plants are tough and bitter. Nip off leaves near stem—tearing them off may damage them.

Roots and tubers: Choose large plants. If difficult to pull up, dig around plant to loosen, then pry out with a sharpened stick.

Fruit and nuts: Pick only ripe, fully colored fruits from large plants. Hard green berries are indigestible. Peel fruits with tough, bitter skins. When nuts are ripe they begin to fall from the tree. Shake the tree or throw a stick to knock other nuts down.

> **CAUTION!** Some seeds and grains contain deadly poisons. Taste, but do not swallow. Carry out edibility test (p. 53) and reject any seed that is unpalatable, bitter, or with a hot, burning taste, unless a positively identified pepper or spice.

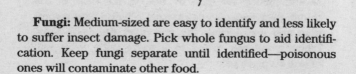

The heads of some grain plants may have enlarged, black bean-like structures in place of normal seeds. These carry a poisonous, hallucinogenic fungal disease that can be lethal. Reject the whole head.

Fungi: Medium-sized are easy to identify and less likely to suffer insect damage. Pick whole fungus to aid identification. Keep fungi separate until identified—poisonous ones will contaminate other food.

IDENTIFYING PLANTS

Only a small selection of plants can be described and illustrated here. Knowledge of even one or two plants that grow widely and at most times of year could make the difference between survival and starvation. Begin by learning these few thoroughly: Temperate zones: dandelion, nettle, dock, plantain; Subtropical and tropical zones: palm, fig, bamboo; Arid and desert zones: mescal, prickly pear, baobab, acacia (not in the Americas); Polar zones: spruce, willow (north), lichens (north and south), many temperate plant species—which grow here in summer; Coastal zones: kelp and laver.

PLANTS TO AVOID

Avoid any plant with milky sap, unless positively identified as safe (e.g., dandelion).

Avoid red plants, unless positively identified.

Avoid fruit which is divided into five segments, unless positively identified as a safe species.

Avoid plants with tiny barbs on stems and leaves: these hooks will irritate mouth and digestive tract.

Avoid old or wilted leaves—some develop deadly toxins when they wilt, e.g., blackberry, raspberry, plum, peach and cherry. All may be eaten safely when young, fresh and dry.

Avoid mature bracken—it destroys vitamin B in the body and can be lethal. Eat only tightly coiled "fiddleheads." All northern temperate ferns are edible when young, but some are too bitter to be palatable and others must have hairy barbs removed before eating: break off young tips, close hand over stalk and draw frond through to remove the "wool."

POISON!
There are two common poisons in the plant world, both easily detectable:
HYDROCYANIC ACID (PRUSSIC ACID): tastes and smells of bitter almonds or peaches. Most notable example is the Cherry Laurel: crush a leaf and memorize the smell. Discard all plants with this smell.
OXALIC ACID: the salts (oxalates) occur in plants such as Wild Rhubarb and Wood Sorrel. Recognizable by the sharp, dry, stinging or burning sensation when applied to the skin or tongue. Discard all plants which fit this description.

ANIMALS FOR FOOD

Your humane instincts must be balanced against the expediencies of survival. Study each species' habits: where it sleeps, what it eats and where it waters. Learn how best to make a kill, what traps to set. The younger the animal, the more lean the meat. Most species put on extra fat to see them through the winter.

FINDING GAME

Tracks and signs: If you can read the subtle signs that animals leave, you will know what hunting/trapping methods to use.

Only large, powerful mammals venture out by day. Most small mammals eat at night, as do those that feed on them. Trails between watering/feeding places and homes are clearest on wet ground, snow and damp sand. Determine the age of the track by its sharpness and moisture content: the clearer it is, the more recent.

In the early morning, check tracks from ground level. If dew and spider's webs have been disturbed, the tracks are fresh. Tunnels through undergrowth and broken twigs along a track will indicate the size of the animal responsible. If trampled leaves have not wilted and broken twigs are green and supple, trail is fresh.

Feedings signs: gnawed bark, discarded food and remains of prey, reveal an animal's presence and suggest bait for traps. For details, see pp. 57–68.

Droppings: Size and quantity indicate type of animal; old droppings will be hard and odorless, fresh ones wet and still smelling. Flies draw attention to them. Break open a dropping to check for clues as to what the animal has been eating, then bait your trap accordingly. Copious bird droppings indicate presence of nesting sites. Seed-eating birds' droppings are small and mostly liquid (indicating water within reasonable range); meat-eaters' pellets contain indigestible parts of prey.

Rootings: Some animals turn over ground in search of insects and tubers. Crumbly, fresh earth means it has been recently dug. A muddy wallow is a sign of pigs.

Scent and smell: Listen to noises and register smells. In cold climates a large animal's breath forms a cloud of condensation which can be seen from afar.

Burrows and dens: Some are easy to find. Hidden ones may be given away by tracks or droppings nearby.

MAMMALS

The following illustrated tracks are not to scale. Most tracks are typical of a family of animals, varying according to species. Where 2 are shown, track 1 is right front, track 2 is right hind.

WEASEL GROUP
Stoats, mink, martens and polecats are all secretive and have sharp, dangerous teeth.

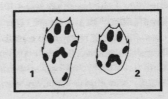

Traps: Spring snares with bait bars and deadfalls. Bait with offal or birds' eggs.

Tracks: Indistinct except in soft ground. Five well-spaced claws and toes, hair on main pad often smudges. Fore and rear prints overlap.

WILD DOGS

Foxes and other species are found from deserts to the Arctic. Wolves are confined to northern wilderness. Canines can be very dangerous. Their superb senses make it pointless to stalk 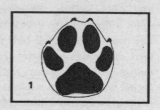 them. Remove anal glands before cooking. Boil thoroughly.

Traps: Snare foxes: try stepped-bait or toggle, bait-release, baited-hole-noose. Minimize human scent.

Tracks and signs: Walk on toes. Print shows four pads and claw tips—outer pad shorter than inner, with large main pad to rear. Elongated, tapering droppings show remains of fur, bones, insects. Fox scent pungent. In soft ground, fox dens can be dug out.

WILD CATS

Occur on all continents except Australia and Antarctica, but not common. Secretive and generally nocturnal. Kills of big cats may be scavenged if unattended, but beware big 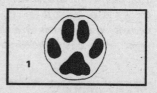 cats. Small cat meat is like rabbit. Stew thoroughly.

Traps: Bait powerful spring snares with offal, blood or meat. Cats have fast reactions and may leap clear of deadfall traps.

Tracks and signs: Walk on toes, claws retracted when walk-

ing (except Cheetah). Droppings elongated, often hidden.
Strong-smelling urine.

MONKEYS AND APES
Confined to tropics, usually live in extended family groups,
often in trees. Even small monkeys can inflict a bad bite.
Intelligent and difficult to stalk. Very edible.
Traps: Perch or baited spring-spear trap, spring snare or hole
noose. Bait with fruit or colorful objects.
Signs: Few take trouble to conceal themselves and most are
noisy.

SEALS
Track shows belly drag in
center. Arrow indicates direction of travel. See p. 30 for
details.

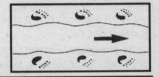

BATS
Found in all except very cold climates. Active at night. Hiber-
nating meat-eaters. Plump fruit bats are especially good
eating. Remove wings and legs, gut and skin like a rabbit.
Vampire bat can transmit rabies: keep well covered if sleep-
ing rough within its range.
Traps: Knock from roosts when sleeping by day.
Signs: Roosting colonies easy to spot. Often in caves.

CATTLE
Live in herds near water.
Bison and other wild cattle
are found in N. America
(protected species), Africa
and S. Asia. Old bulls are
particularly dangerous.

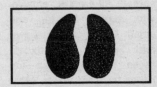

Traps: Powerful snares, spring traps and deadfalls.
Tracks and signs: Heavy, two distinct hoofmarks, narrow at top, bulbous at rear. Droppings are like cow pats. They make excellent fuel.

WILD SHEEP AND GOATS

Sheep tend to live in small flocks in inaccessible places. Goats are even more sure-footed than sheep and almost impossible to approach.

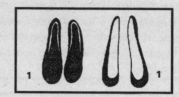

Traps: Snares or spring snares on trails. In rocky areas natural obstructions are ideal for deadfalls.
Tracks and signs: Cloven hooves, two slender pointed marks not joined, tip splayed in sheep, sometimes in goats. Illustration: domestic sheep (left), chamois (right). Globular droppings like domestic sheep.

DEER AND ANTELOPES

Deer, found in well-wooded country on every continent except Australia, vary from the moose to tiny forest deer of the tropics. Antelopes and gazelles are equally varied and widespread. All are shy, elusive, with superb hearing and smell. Most active at dawn and dusk, and—except those in arid areas—are never far from water. Meat

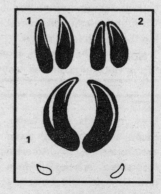

smokes well. Use hides and antlers. Their horns are weapons and can gouge and stab.

Traps: Snare or deadfall small types. Leg spring snares spear traps and deadfalls for larger. Bait with offal.

Tracks and signs: Cloven hooves form two oblongs. Reindeer marks are rounded. The illustration shows, in relative scale, roe deer front and hind track (top); and reindeer (bottom).

Note dew-claw impression on reindeer track. When walking, front and rear prints overlap; and when running they are spaced. Droppings oblong to round pellets, usually in clumps.

Look for scrapes on saplings, nibbled and frayed bark. Also long scratches where antlers have been rubbed.

WILD PIGS

Some have thick hair, and all are pig-shaped with snouts and tusks. They are hard to stalk—listen for snores and creep up on sleeping ones! Meat must be well boiled.Their tusks 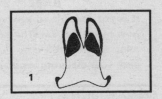 inflict severe injury, often dangerously close to femoral artery on the upper leg. Beware!

Traps: Strong spring snares, deadfall, pig spear traps.

Tracks and signs: Cloven hooves leave deer-like marks. Droppings are often shapeless, never long, firm or tapering. Look for ground disturbed by mudwallows or rooting.

RABBITS AND HARES

Rabbits are widespread and easy to catch. Most live in burrows, often in large numbers and using well-worn runs—the places to set snares. Hares do not live in burrows and tend not to have regular runs.

Traps: Simple snares. A spring snare will lessen the chance of your meal being stolen by other prey.

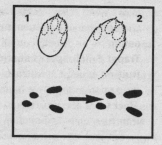

Tracks and signs: Hairy soles leave little detail on soft ground. Combination of long hind and short front feet is distinctive. Hares have 5 toes on front feet, but inner is short and seldom leaves print. Hind foot narrower, 4-toed. Rabbit similar but smaller. Droppings small, hard round pellets. Bark nibbled at bottom of trees leaving two incisor marks. Rabbits thump a warning.

RABBIT STARVATION

It is not possible to survive on rabbit alone, no matter how many you eat. The body needs minerals and vitamins which rabbit does not provide: make sure to balance your diet with vegetation.

SMALL RODENTS

Rats, mice, guinea pigs, cavies, capybara, copyu and other members of the rodent family may be tempted into cage traps—most species are too small to snare. Tracks of different kinds are not easy to distinguish. Rats carry disease. When gutting, take care not to rupture the innards. Cook thoroughly.

SQUIRRELS AND PRAIRIE DOGS

Occur everywhere except Australasia and the Poles, hibernating in cold areas. Alert and nimble, most are active by day and night.

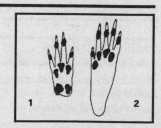

Beware of their sharp teeth—they are savage in defense. Ground-living varieties make burrows. Most are excellent eating.

Traps: Small spring snares attached to bait bars. Use split fruit or an egg to attract. For tree squirrels set 5 cm (2 in) loop snares on a pole leaned against a trunk.

Tracks and signs: Chewed bark, gnawed nuts, cones beneath a tree or an untidy nest of twigs.

KANGAROOS

With wallabies and other relatives, limited to Australia. Large kinds can strike a powerful blow with hind feet. Most active at night. Edibility fair, but difficult to catch.

Traps: Deadfalls, spring snares.

Tracks and signs: Two prints resembling giant rabbit tracks (front legs not used for locomotion).

OPOSSUMS

Small nocturnal scavengers of S. America and USA. Similar, unrelated animals found in Australasia.

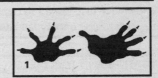

Traps: Bait with fruit, eggs, etc. Very inquisitive.

RACCOONS

Cat-sized nocturnal animals with bushy banded tail and black mask. Found widely in N. America.

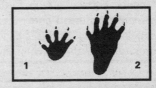

Traps: Bait a spring snare.

CAMELS

Range wild in desert country. Can spit and inflict powerful

bites. They require a very powerful spear or projectile weapon.

REPTILES

CROCODILES AND ALLIGATORS

Found in most subtropical and tropical areas. Avoid large ones. In areas where they live, always assume they are about for they can lie unseen underwater. Their tails can inflict a scything blow almost as damaging as their teeth. Tail meat is very tasty.

Traps: Set by water for small crocs only, or catch on line with stick wedged in bait to lodge in gullet. Kill with a sharp blow between the eyes.

LIZARDS

Some are venomous. Most are timid, but big iguanas and monitors can inflict a bad bite and have powerful claws. Small ones move fast, but try to catch by the tail. Can sometimes be trapped in a pit or may fall into a solar still.

TURTLES AND TORTOISES

Most live in water, emerging to lay eggs, but a few are terrestrial. Net or drag them from the water. On land use a stick to turn them on their backs. Keep out of the way of jaws and flippers. Kill with a blow to the head. Cut through belly and discard guts, head and neck. Best boiled. Very rich, eat in small amounts. Tortoises can retract heads—stab, then roast ungutted in embers. When shell splits they are ready.

AMPHIBIANS

Frogs are all edible, but skins may be poisonous so remove before cooking. Active at night near water. Dazzle with a light and club them.

Toads have warty skins and may be found far from water. Most have highly toxic skin—do not eat it.

SNAKES

Do not tackle poisonous or large ones. Use a forked stick to pin it down just behind head. Strike back of head with another stick. Tree snakes can be clubbed and knocked to ground. Club again to make sure!

Never pick up or get close to a snake until you are sure it is dead. Some can feign death convincingly.

BIRDS

All birds are edible, but some taste better than others. Game birds are good to eat but well camouflaged and wary. Birds of prey must be boiled thoroughly.

Traps: Cage traps, deadfalls and spring snares can be used for birds that take bait. Nooses on branches may catch roosting birds. In wooded areas, site traps in clearings or by riverbanks. Small birds are easy to catch or lime and can be attracted by bait. A crude dummy owl will lure small birds.

Tracks and signs: In desert and on snow, tracks may help to locate birds hiding in close cover. Droppings may indicate a night roost. Alarm calls may help locate other animals.

Autumn molt: Birds molt completely in autumn and are unable to fly more than short distances. Ducks, geese and game birds are easy to catch at this time.

Nests: Eggs are easily available from ground nesters. Approach colonies carefully—crawling not walking—to get within stone-throwing or clubbing distance. Some guard nests tenaciously. Be prepared for attack.

Flightless birds: Large birds such as ostriches should be treated with caution: they can deliver powerful kicks.

INSECTS

Rich in fat, protein and carbohydrates. Overcome your squeamishness. Look in nooks and crannies of trees and in moist shady spots. Look for beetle grubs—pale in color with three short legs—on trees with peeling bark and in decaying stumps. Collect living specimens. Avoid any that look sick or dead, have a bad smell or produce a rash when handled. Take care: scorpions, spiders and snakes also shelter in nooks and crannies.

Most are edible raw, but more palatable cooked. Boiling is safest. Alternatively, roast by placing on hot stones or in the embers of a fire. Remove legs and wings from larger insects—fine hairs can irritate the digestive tract. To eat a hairy caterpillar, squeeze to extract the innards, do not eat skin. Take armor casing off beetles.

Small insects can be mashed to a paste and cooked or dried to a powder, then used to thicken other foods such as soups or stews.

Do not gather insects feeding on carrion, refuse or dung—they may carry infection. Avoid grubs found on the underside of leaves, they often secrete toxins. Use as fish bait. Brightly colored insects and caterpillars are usually poisonous. Large beetles often have powerful jaws.

TERMITES

Found in warm climates. Most eat only vegetation but big ones have sharp jaws and will bite anything. Termites build mounds up to several feet high. Break off pieces and dunk in water to force termites out. A piece of the nest placed on embers will produce a fragrant smoke that will keep mosquitoes away. When fishing, suspend a piece of nest above a pool; termites falling from it will be good bait. Alternatively, insert a twig into the nest and gently withdraw it. Termites will bite it and hang on—but you won't catch very many.

Remove wings from large termites before boiling, frying or roasting. The eggs are nutritious too.

BEES, WASPS AND HORNETS

Bees are edible throughout life cycle. Honey is easily digestible and highly nutritious, but difficult to collect. Nests are found in hollow trees or caves, or under an overhanging rock. Strike at night: make a torch from a bundle of grass and hold it close to the entrance so nest fills with smoke. Then seal hole. That kills bees, providing an immediate meal and a supply of honey.

Remove wings, legs and sting, before eating. Boiling or roasting improves flavor. Comb may be eaten, and wax used to waterproof clothing or make candles. In some places, there is a slight risk that honey may contain concentrations of plant poisons. Smell will be one guide, but use edibility test given for plants.

Wasps and hornets are dangerous. Hornets sting on sight and the pain is extreme. Search for a safer meal.

ANTS

Most ants have a stinging bite. Some fire formic acid. They must be cooked for at least six minutes to destroy the poison. They are then quite safe to eat.

LOCUSTS, CRICKETS AND GRASSHOPPERS

All have plump bodies and muscled legs. Swat with a leafy branch or clothing. Remove wings, antennae and legs. Eat raw or roast to kill parasites.

SNAILS, SLUGS AND WORMS

Must be eaten fresh after special preparation.

Snails are found in fresh water, saltwater and on land. Rich in proteins and minerals. Ones with brightly colored shells may be poisonous. Sea snails should be left alone unless positively identified. Starve snails or slugs for a few days, or feed only on herbs and safe greens so they can excrete poisons. Place in a saltwater solution to clear out guts. Boil for 10 minutes, adding herbs for flavor.

Worms are high in protein. Starve them for a day, or squeeze them between fingers to clear muck out. Can be sun or force-dried—leave them on a hot stone—then ground into powder to thicken other food.

DANGERS

The numerous diseases carried by mosquitoes, ticks and other insects, and the unseen dangers of parasites you may pick up from food or water, and various water-borne diseases, are much more serious than attacks by animals.

DANGEROUS CONFRONTATIONS

Attacks by animals are rare, but large animals can be dangerous. Keep out of their way. Use self-control, do not unintentionally provoke the animal to attack.

If you come face to face with a large animal, freeze. Slowly back off and talk in a calm manner. Avoid sudden movements and remember animals can smell fear—many a hunter has fouled his breeches and given himself away. Do your best to calm yourself.

If an animal appears to charge it may be that you are blocking its escape route. Move out of the way.

If an animal gives chase (or you haven't the nerve to freeze or sidestep), zig-zag when you run. Some animals—e.g., rhinos—have poor eyesight or charge in a straight line.

Nocturnal predators have excellent night vision but

their color vision is poor. They cannot see stationery objects well. Freeze if it hasn't already seen you.

Shouting and making a commotion may put off a predator.

Taking to a tree is the last resort, you may be treed for a long time. Don't choose a thorn tree if you can help it, you may get badly scratched and become trapped on an extremely painful perch.

TRAPS AND TRAPPING

It is easier to trap than to hunt small prey. Choice of baits and site is important. Food may be scarce, but a little used as bait may bring rewards. Be patient and give the traps time. Animals will be wary until they get used to them—that is when they will run into them.

Regular checking is essential. Leaving a trap line unchecked will prolong an animal's pain and increase the risk of your catch struggling free—animals will bite off a limb to escape—or being poached by predators.

Establish as large a trap line as you can. Collect game and reset traps, repairing as necessary and removing any that are repeatedly unfruitful. Accept a proportion of failures, but if the bait has gone without the trap being fired it is an indication that the trigger mechanism is too tight or the bait insecurely fixed. Check both when you reset the trap.

Set traps on game trails or runs. Look for natural bottlenecks, e.g., where the track passes under an obstruction. Do not place a trap close to an animal's lair—it will be alert to anything unusual close to home.

When alarmed, animals panic and take the shortest route to cover. That is when the crudest and most obvious traps will be successful.

MANGLE   STRANGLE   DANGLE   TANGLE
Deadfalls mangle. Snares strangle. Saplings can take
the prey in the air—it dangles.The higher the sapling
the more effectively it lifts the animal. A net tangles.
Some traps combine two or more of these principles.

RULES FOR TRAPS

1 **Avoid disturbing environment:** Don't tread on game trail,
leave no sign that you have been there.

2 **Hide scent:** Handle traps as little as possible and wear
gloves if you can. Do not set a trap of pinewood in a wood
of hazel. Mask human scents by exposing snare to campfire smoke.

3 **Camouflage:** Hide freshly cut ends of wood with mud.
Cover ground snares to blend in naturally.

4 **Make them strong:** An ensnared animal will fight for its
life. Any weakness in the traps will soon be exposed.

Snares

Snares can be improvised from string, rope, twine or,
ideally, nonferrous wire with a running eye at one end
through which the other end passes before being anchored
to a stake, rock or tree. A snare is a free-running noose
which catches small game by the throat and large game
around the legs.

*A wire snare can be supported off the
ground on twigs, which can
also be used to keep a
suspended string noose
open. Set the snare
a hand's length
from an
obstruction to
trap rabbits.*

USING A SIMPLE SNARE FOR SMALL ANIMALS
Make the loop a fist-width wide
Set it four fingers above the ground and a hand's width
from an obstruction
Anchor securely. Support loop with twigs if necessary.

When constructing a snare under tension, use a sapling
to lift the game off the ground. The trap is then more effective: the animal is less able to struggle and predators can't
get at it. Hazel is ideal for this.

Spring snare: Good for rabbits and foxes. Situate on
trail by a natural bottleneck caused by dead fall or rock.

*Cut notch in trigger bar (a) to fit notch in upright (b). Drive upright into
ground. Attach snare to trigger bar and use cord to sapling to keep
tension. Bar disengages, lifting game in air.*

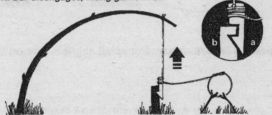

Baited spring snare: ideal for medium-sized prey.

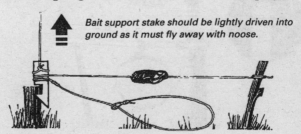

*Bait support stake should be lightly driven into
ground as it must fly away with noose.*

Baited spring leg snare: Push prongs of a natural fork of wood (or 2 sticks tied together) into the ground. The line from a bent sapling is tied to a toggle and to the snare; toggle is then passed under fork. Bait is attached to a separate bar. Ideal for large game: deer, big cats, bear. For deer, bait with blood or scent glands to arouse its curiosity.

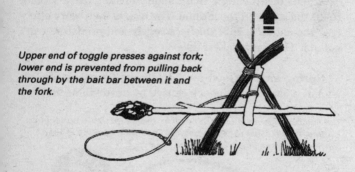

Upper end of toggle presses against fork; lower end is prevented from pulling back through by the bait bar between it and the fork.

Spring tension snare: For small animals. Site on trail.

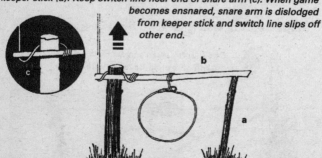

Switch line secures one end of snare arm (b) while the other rests on keeper stick (a). Keep switch line near end of snare arm (c). When game becomes ensnared, snare arm is dislodged from keeper stick and switch line slips off other end.

Trapeze spring snare: Use to cover two game trails in open country.

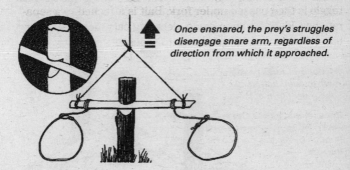

Once ensnared, the prey's struggles disengage snare arm, regardless of direction from which it approached.

Roller spring snare: Good for rabbits and foxes.

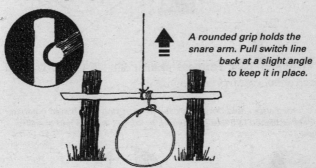

A rounded grip holds the snare arm. Pull switch line back at a slight angle to keep it in place.

A wide area can be covered using several snares on long horizontal bar. Use where game trail widens.

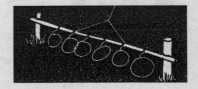

Platform trap: Site in a small depression on game trail. Place snares on platforms on either side. When platform is depressed, trigger bar is released and game held by the leg. Ideal for deer, big cats, bear.

Platform of sticks or stiff bark rests on bottom bar. Upper bar fits in notches.

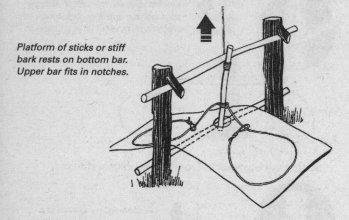

Stepped bait release snare: Site in clearings. Will catch small carnivores and pigs.

Two forked sticks hold down a cross-bar engaging with baited notched upright (attached to a line in tension), holding it in place and carrying snares.

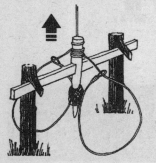

Retaining bar should be squared off to fit square-cut notch on the bait stick.

Deadfall traps

These traps work on the principle that when the bait is taken a weight falls on the prey.

> ☠️ Large versions of traps can be dangerous for humans. Toggle release and deadfall traps are easily set off accidentally. In a survival situation ensure that everyone know where the traps are. In survival practice keep people away from them and never leave a trap set up at the end of an exercise.

Setting a deadfall trap is risky. You cannot do it on your own. Keep the mechanism to the side of the trail, away from the dropping weight. Balance is critical—you are unlikely to get it right the first time.

Toggle trip-release deadfall: A mechanism similar to the toggle-release snare, but here the release bar keeping the toggle in position presses one end of the toggle upward. A line from the toggle passes over a tree limb to support a weight (e.g., logs) above the trail. A trip line runs aboveground beneath the suspended weight to a securing point.

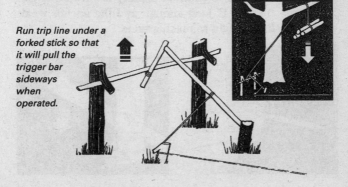

Run trip line under a forked stick so that it will pull the trigger bar sideways when operated.

Balance log: A forked stick, its ends sharpened to dislodge easily, one fork baited, supports one end of a crossbar. The other end rests on a fixed support, held there by the heavy logs or rock with rests on the bar. The trap collapses when the bait is taken.

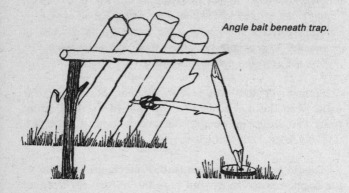

Angle bait beneath trap.

Deadfall trap: A weight suspended over the trail pulls the line carrying it against a retaining bar held by short pegs secured in a tree trunk at slightly downward angle. Make sure the line is long enough and the anchor weak enough to allow weight to reach ground.

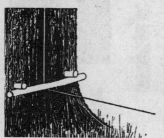
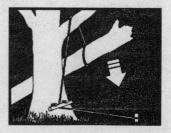

Figure 4 deadfall trap: Balance a horizontal bait bar at right angles to an upright with a locking bar which supports a weight, positioned over bait, pivoted on sharpened tip of upright.

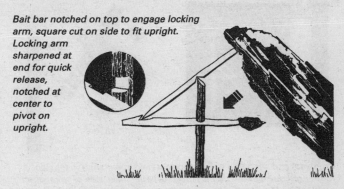

Bait bar notched on top to engage locking arm, square cut on side to fit upright. Locking arm sharpened at end for quick release, notched at center to pivot on upright.

Spear traps

These traps can be lethal to humans. Always stand behind the spear when setting and mark with signs to warn humans the trap is there. Except in a survival situation, never leave spear traps set and unsupervised.

Deadfall spear trap:

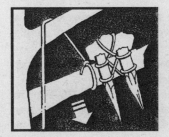

Same mechanism as deadfall trap (p. 76, but rocks add weight and sharpened sticks deliver a stabbing blow.

Spring spear trap: A springy shaft with a spear attached is held taut over the trail. A slip ring made of smooth material attached to a trip wire acts as release.

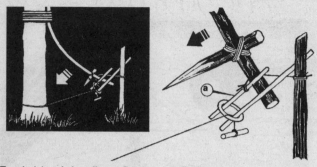

Toggle (a) and short line to fixed upright hold spear shaft in tension. A further rod through the ring is tensed between near side of spear shaft and far face of upright, securing the trap.

Bird traps

Nets: Stretch a fine net between trees where birds roost. Alternatively, a fine twine crisscrossed between trees across their flight path will damage birds which fly into it.

Bird lime: Boil holly leaves and any starchy grain in water; simmer until you have a gooey mess. Spread this on branches and perching places. Birds will get stuck in it when they alight.

Suspended snares: Hang a line of snares across a stream a little above water level. This works best among reeds and rushes.

Baited hooks: Bury fish hooks in fruit or other food. The hook gets caught in the bird's throat.

Noose sticks: Tie fine nooses 1.25–2.5 cm (½–1 in) in diameter in horsehair. Place stick in roosting or nesting spot with nooses uppermost. Do not remove as soon as the first bird becomes entangled—it will attract others into the trap.

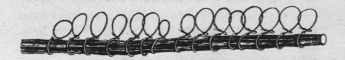

Figure 4 trap: This mechanism (*see Figure 4 deadfall p. 77*) can be used with a cage made from a pyramid of sticks tied together and balanced over the bait. For small birds, lay all sticks in position, then lay another two sticks, the same length as the bottom ones, on top and tie them tightly to the bottom layer, tight enough to keep all the others in place. Larger animals are stronger; for them each stick must be individually tied.

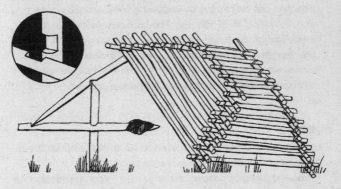

Running noose: Use a noose attached to a long pole to pull down roosting birds. Go to roosting site on a bright night. Slip noose over bird, tighten as you pull.

Stalking waterfowl: Get up close by getting into water and camouflaging your head with reeds or vegetation. Cautiously approach the nesting area, bearing in mind that birds can be ferocious in self-defense.

Where large gourds are available, make holes on one side to see and breathe through, then place over head. Throw several other gourds into water to prepare birds. The hunter then floats with current among birds, grabs them from below and strangles them underwater.

Pit trap: Find or dig a hole 90 cm (3 ft) deep in an area where ground-feeding birds are common. The pit's width depends on the type of birds. Spread grain or bait around the hole and more concentratedly inside it. First taking the bait around the hole, birds will enter it to get more. Rush them: in their panic they are unable to spread their wings sufficiently to take off from inside the hole.

SEAGULLS

Seagulls can be caught by wrapping food around a stone and throwing it in the air. The gull swallows the bait while still on the wing, gulps down the stone with it, and the weight change causes it to crash. Obviously this is a technique for use over land rather than at sea. Be ready to dispatch the bird as soon as it hits the ground.

HUNTING

Keen observation and a knowledge of animals make it easier to find prey and to take advantage of terrain.

Proceed quietly. Move slowly and stop regularly. To avoid stumbles and reduce noise, carry your weight on the rear foot, testing the next step with the toes before transferring your weight. Hunt against the wind.

If an animal catches a glimpse of you, freeze. It may be more curious than frightened. Remain still until the animal looks away or continues feeding.

Hunt at first light, moving uphill, and return to camp in the afternoon. Tracks are easier to read moving uphill; thermal currents build up with the heat of day and carry scents upward, so by returning downhill the scent of game reaches you before yours reaches them. If you must hunt in the evening, go out at least an hour before dusk so your eyes can develop night vision, but your prey will probably see better than you do.

Get as close as you can to your prey and take steady aim at a point just to the back of the front shoulder. A hit here will drop most animals instantly.

If an animal drops, wait 5 minutes before moving in. Stand back and observe. If hurt, loss of blood will weaken it and when you do approach it will be unable to bolt. If a wounded animal moves away, wait 15 minutes before following, otherwise it will run all day.

Avoid large animals unless really confident of a first-shot kill—or you could end up becoming the hunted and not the hunter.

WEAPONS
Bow and arrow

The most effective of improvised weapons: easy to make, it takes only a short time to become proficient.

A well-seasoned wood is best for the bow. Long-term survivors should put wood aside to season. Tension in unseasoned wood is short-lived, so make several bows and change as soon as one loses its spring.

Yew is ideal, but hickory, juniper, oak, white elm, cedar, ironwood, birch, willow and hemlock (the tree) are good alternatives.

Making the stave:

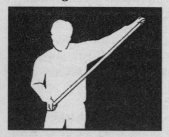

Select a supple wand. To determine correct length: hold one end of stave at the hip with right hand, reach sideways with left hand and mark extent of your reach as length of bow.

Shaping the bow:

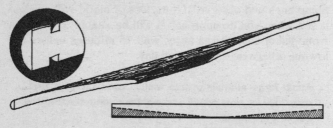

Stave must be 5 cm (2 in) wide at center, tapering to 1.5 cm (⅝ in) at ends. Make notch about 1.25 cm (½ in) from ends (a) to take bowstring. Remove bark if you wish. Once whittled into shape, rub bow with oil or animal fat.

Fitting the string: Cut rawhide to 3 mm (⅛ in) wide or use string, or twisted fibers from nettle stems to make bowstring. If bow has lots of give, use shorter string. String should be under only slight tension—the main tension is added when you pull it back to shoot.

Secure string to bow with round turn and two half hitches at each end. If wood is unseasoned, release one end when bow is not in use to relax its tension.

Making arrows: Use straight wood—birch is best. Make arrows 60 cm (2 ft) long, 6 mm (¼ in) wide. They must be as straight and smooth as possible.

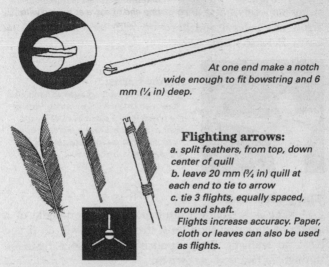

At one end make a notch wide enough to fit bowstring and 6 mm (¼ in) deep.

Flighting arrows:
a. split feathers, from top, down center of quill
b. leave 20 mm (¾ in) quill at each end to tie to arrow
c. tie 3 flights, equally spaced, around shaft.
Flights increase accuracy. Paper, cloth or leaves can also be used as flights.

Arrow heads: The arrow itself can be sharpened and hardened in fire, but a tip of tin or flint is better. Split end of shaft, insert arrow head and bind tightly with wet sinews—they dry hard, securing head firmly.

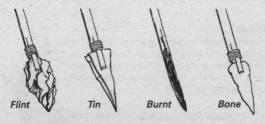

Flint   Tin   Burnt   Bone

For details of how to make flint arrowheads see p. 140.

Archery technique: Fit arrow into bowstring. Raise center of bow to eye level. Hold bow just below arrow, extending arm forward. Keep bow arm locked and draw string smoothly back across the front of your body, with arrow at eye-level and lined up with target. Sight along arrow. Release string.

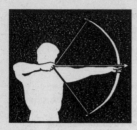

Arrow burns:
Arrow flights rubbing against hand and cheek can cause friction burns. Protect the cheek with a piece of cloth pulled tight to the face. Wear a leather mitten or fit a leather guard between fingers and wrist to protect hand.

Sling and shot
A sling is a simple leather pouch in the middle of a length of thong or rope (any strong fabric will do if you have no leather). Attach pouch as one piece threaded through, or two tied or sewn on.

Slingshot technique:
Use round smooth pebbles 2 cm (¾ in) across. Swing the sling above the head in a circle lined up on your target. Release one end of rope and ammunition should fly at target. Experiment with sling length to achieve accuracy and distance.

Catapult
Take a strong, pliable forked twig (hazel is ideal) and a piece of elastic material (innertube from a tire or elastic from clothing). Thread or sew a pouch into the center of the elastic, tie ends to each side of fork. Use stones as missiles.

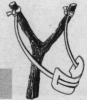

Load several pebbles at a time when using sling or catapult against birds.

Spears

A straight staff 1.8 m (6 ft) is ideal for a jabbing spear; 90 cm (3 ft) is best for throwing. Make a spear thrower from a piece of wood half that length to improve accuracy.

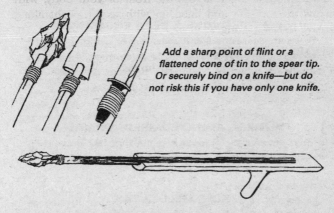

Add a sharp point of flint or a flattened cone of tin to the spear tip. Or securely bind on a knife—but do not risk this if you have only one knife.

Spear thrower: Take a tree limb twice the width of spear, with branch stump to serve as handle. Split down center, using knife as wedge. Gouge out a cleanly cut groove along most of upper face of thrower. Leave a solid portion as a buffer to add thrust.

Hold spear at shoulder level and aim at target, bringing holder sharply forward then downward.

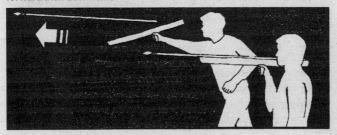

THE DANGERS OF HUNTING

Few animals will attack except in self-defense, but don't camp on a trail or near an animal watering spot.

DON'T PROVOKE A BEAR ENCOUNTER

Bears are scavengers and will come to camps in search of food. Don't get close or try to catch them. A bear can easily kill a human. Use noise to drive them off—the same goes for other scavengers, e.g., hyenas.

INJURED AND CORNERED ANIMALS

Most animals try to escape when hurt. By preventing them from doing so you are forcing them to fight.

KEEP WELL CLEAR

Crocodiles and alligators should be given a wide berth. Large horned animals may wound you before you can reach your weapon. Many animals, not just those with hooves, have deadly kicks—including ostriches.

BITES

Many small animals have sharp teeth and will attack ferociously. Chimpanzees and other monkeys can be very bad-tempered. Thoroughly cleanse any bites: they may cause tetanus. Some animals carry rabies.

SNAKES AND STINGING INSECTS

Get used to checking clothing, bedding and equipment for reptiles and insects. If you awake to find one in your sleeping bag, move gently and calmly to get rid of them or to free yourself.

HANDLING THE KILL

Before approaching, check that your prey is dead. Use a spear or tie your knife to a long stick and stab a large animal in its main muscles and neck. Loss of blood will weaken it, allowing you to move in and club the head.

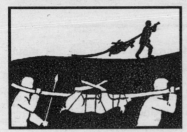

Two people can carry a large animal tied to a bough. Place pole along belly and use clove hitch around each pair of legs. Lash animal to pole and finish with clove hitch around pole. If it has horns, tie these up out of the way or cut off head.

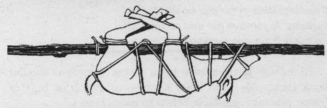

Butcher game on the trap line. Other meat eaters will be attracted and may become trapped. Use entrails to bait traps. Only carry to camp what you can manage without exertion: in camp it will only attract flies and scavengers. Cache remainder for collection later.

HIDING THE KILL

Suspend a carcass from a bough, out of reach from the branch. A cache in the crook of a tree will keep meat away from ground predators but will still be accessible to climbing predators. Where vultures are present the cache will be impossible to protect.

☠ HEALTH HAZARDS—DISEASED ANIMALS
All animals have lymph glands in their cheeks. If large and discolored, the animal is ill. Any animal that is distorted or discolored about the head should be boiled and care taken in preparation: cover cuts or sores in your skin when handling meat.

PREPARING THE KILL
Waste nothing: make use of parts you cannot eat. Set about preparing the kill in four stages:

Bleeding: Essential if meat is to keep. Blood is valuable food, rich in vitamins and minerals, including salt, that are essential to survival. Keep cool in covered vessel.
Skinning: Hide or fur can be used.
Gutting: To remove gut and recover offal.
Jointing: Produces suitable cuts for cooking.

Bleeding: Hang animal head down. Tie ropes around hock (not ankle) and hoist it up to a branch or build a frame, placing receptacle below to catch blood.

For a frame: drive strong posts into ground and lash firmly to make A-frames. Rest horizontal bar on top.

Bleed animal by cutting jugular vein or carotid artery in its neck. When animal is hanging, these will bulge clearly. Make cut either behind ears—stab in line with ears to pierce vein on both sides of head at same time—or lower down in V of neck, before artery branches. Unless you have a stiletto knife, the latter is best. Cutting throat from ear to ear risks contamination of blood with contents of stomach. It is important to bleed pigs thoroughly if the meat is to be saved.

Skinning: While flesh is still warm, remove any scent glands (deer have them behind knee of rear legs; felines on either side of anus). Remove testicles of males. To remove hide, cut through skin as shown by broken lines on illustration below.

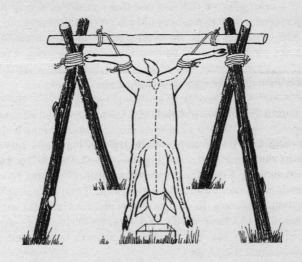

1 Make ring around rear legs just above knee.
2 Cut around forelegs in same place.
3 Cut down inside of rear legs to crotch; cut circle around genitals.
4 Extend cut down center of body to neck. Do not cut into stomach and digestive organs. Lift skin as you go, slip in the knife, sharp edge outward, and cut along. Draw knife slowly down, cutting away from body.
5 Cut down inside of forelegs.

Now ease skin of rear legs from the flesh. Use the knife as little as possible. Roll skin outward, fur inside itself, and pull down. When back legs are clear, cut around tail. Insert hand down back of carcass and use fingers to separate flesh from skin. Next, peel skin from front legs. Separate the single piece of hide from the neck with a strong twist of the head. Cut through remaining tissues.

If working alone, lay carcass down a slope, scoop an impression in the ground to hold the collecting vessel.

Skin small animals by making incision over stomach (do not pierce organs). Insert thumbs and pull out. Free legs and twist head off. If you have no knife, snap off lower part of leg and use the sharp edge to cut skin.

Gutting: Remove gut and offal from suspended carcass by pinching abdomen as high as possible and making a slit big enough to take two fingers in the pinched flesh. Insert fingers and use them as a guide for the knife to cut upward, then downward, using hand to prevent gut from spilling. Cut down as far as breastbone. Then let gut spill out, hanging down. Remove kidneys and liver. Cut through membrane to chest cavity and remove heart, lungs and windpipe. You should be able to see daylight through anus—check it is clear.

Jointing meat: Large animals can be quartered by first splitting down backbone, then cutting each side between tenth and eleventh rib. Hindquarters contain steaks (rump and fillet) and choicer cuts. Forequarter meat is more stringy and needs slow cooking to make it tender. Cuts vary according to the kind of animal.

OFFAL

Liver: Eat as soon as possible. Little cooking is required. Remove bile bladder in the center with care, don't allow it to taint meat. Avoid mottled or white-spotted liver.

Stomach: Tripe is easy to digest. Remove stomach contents (good invalid food, as it is already broken down, so boil lightly), wash tripe and simmer slowly with herbs.

Kidneys: Boil with herbs. White fat surrounding them (suet) can be rendered down to use in pemmican; see p. 137.

Lungs (lights): Do not eat if mottled with black and white spots. If pink and blemish free, boil, or use for bait.

Heart: Roast, or use to liven up a stew.

Intestines: Ideal sausage skins: turn inside out and wash. Then boil well. Mix equal proportions of fat and meat, then stir in blood. Stuff the skins with this mixture and boil well. If smoked, sausages keep for a long time.

Sweetbreads (pancreas): Boil or roast.

Tail: Skin and boil to make soup.

Feet: Clean well, then boil to make stew.

Head: Large animal heads are meaty. Boil tongue to make it tender and skin before eating. Brain will make brawn and provide a solution to cure hides. Boil whatever is left, or the whole head with small animals.

Bones: Boil for soup—marrow is rich in vitamins. They can also be made into tools.

Hanging: Eat offal as soon as possible, but rest of meat is better hung to make it tender and to kill parasites. In moderate temperatures, leave carcass hanging for 2–3 days. In hot climates, preserve or cook at once.

Preparing sheep-like animals: Follow instructions for large animals, then split in two down center of spine. Remove rear leg (cut through the joint) and front leg. Cut off neck and loose flesh below ribs. Cut between ribs and vertebrae. Preserve the fillet, found in the small of the back.

Preparing pig: Do not skin. Gut, then place over hot embers and scrape hair off (loosen it with water just hotter than your hand can bear). Boil, to kill parasites.

Preparing reptiles: Discard internal organs. Cook in skin. Cut off head well down, behind poison sacs; open vent to neck, keeping blade turned outward—don't pierce innards. Skewer to suspend. Ease the skin down toward the tail.

Preparing birds: To kill, stretch the neck and cut throat, or cut just under the tongue to sever main artery. Hang head-down to bleed. Meat-eaters harbor parasites, so handle them as little as possible. Pluck while body is still warm. Hot water will loosen the feathers (except those of waterfowl). Make incision from vent to tail, insert hand and draw out guts. Retain heart and kidneys. Cut off head and feet. Boil meat-eaters and old birds; young ones can be roasted on spit or in oven. Leave skins on and eat them.

FISH AND FISHING

Fish contain protein, vitamins and fats. They differ widely in size, eating habits and diet, but all can be attracted and caught with appropriate bait. Angling is not the most effective method of catching fish—the night line and gill net will give better results—but if you have plenty of time it is a pleasurable pastime.

Where to fish: If it is hot and the water is low, fish retreat to deep, shaded waters. In cold weather, they seek shallow spots where the sun warms the water. At any time, fish like to shelter under banks and rocks.

When a river is in flood, fish in slack water, e.g., on the outside of a bend or in a small tributary.

When to fish: Leave lines out overnight and check them just before first light. If a storm is imminent, fish before it breaks. Fishing is poor after heavy rain.

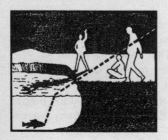

Image refraction:
Fish can see more on the bank than you think. Sit or kneel when fishing, so you are less likely to be in vision. Keep back from the edge and try to keep your shadow off the water.

Indications of fish feeding: Fish are likely to take bait when you see them jumping out of the water. Clear ring ripples breaking on the surface are another sign. Where lots of little fish are darting about, they may be being pursued by a larger predatory fish.

ANGLING

You can improvise hooks from all kinds of materials. Here (from left to right) are a pin, a thorn, a bunch of thorns, nails, bone and wood.

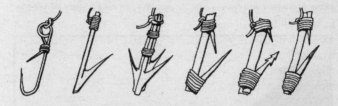

Large hooks will catch large fish, but small ones catch large and small. A rod is not essential (you can fish with a handline) but it makes it easier to land fish and cast away from the bank.

Angling without hooks:
Eels and catfish swallow without biting. To catch them, tie a blob of worms on a line (a) and pull them out as soon as bait is taken. A small sharp piece of wood attached to the end of the line, and held flat along it by the bait (b) will, when the bait is swallowed, open out across the gullet of the fish (c).

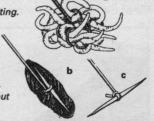

Bait: Fish are more likely to take bait native to their water: berries that overhang it, insects that breed in it. Examine stomach contents of your first catch for clues.

Using Floats and Weights

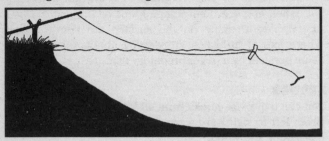

A small floating object attached to the line, visible from the bank, will show you when you have a bite. Its position will help control where the line descends.

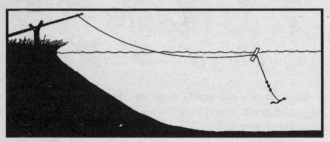

Small weights between float and hook stop the line trailing along the water or too near the surface, while leaving the hook itself in movement. Your survival kit includes a small split lead shot. Slip the groove along the line and squeeze to fit tightly.

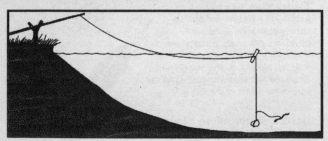

To get a deeper hook position, extend line to a weight below the hook.

Any suitable bait, scattered on water, will attract fish. Put the same bait on your hook to catch them. Suspend a termite or ant nest over water and the falling insects will prove an irresistible draw to fish.

Spinning: Fish will attack a shiny object drawn through water: try coins, buttons, tin, or buckles. Thread a propeller shape to a piece of wire and it will spin with the current. Attach your hook to the end of the spindle.

Artificial bait:

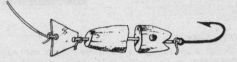

Feathers tied to a hook with thread can simulate a fly. Try to make lures move like live bait: carve a small jointed fish out of wood (hazel is best for cutting through), thread the segments and decorate with color or glitter.

Live bait: Cover hook completely with worms, insects, maggots, or small fish. A hook can be placed through a small fish or grasshopper without killing it. The distressed movement of the bait will attract fish.

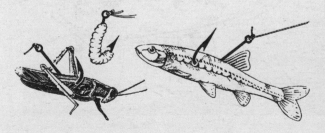

Night lines:

Weight one end of a line and attach worm-baited hooks at intervals. Anchor free end securely on bank. Put this out overnight—use in daytime too, but change worms regularly because fresh wriggling ones attract more attention.

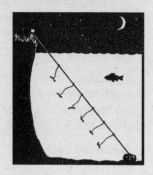

Otter board:

To fish farther than you can cast a line, make a board with a moveable pivoted rudder. Set a bar at front end of rudder and attach two control lines. Suspend baited hooks below. Float board out into lake. If winds are favorable, mount a sail, but first add a keel: gouge holes to fix dowel supports and tie on a flat stone (not so big as to conflict with the rudder). Undue movement of the board indicates a bite.

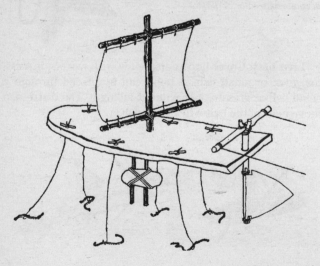

Jigging or snagging:

When you can see fish but they are not taking bait, tie several hooks to a pole and lower it into water. Suspend a bright object 20 cm (8 in) above the pole, and when fish go to inspect it, pull hooks up sharply to catch them.

FISH TRAPS

In shallow streams build a channel of sticks or rocks that fish can swim into but not turn around in (arrows here indicate the current).

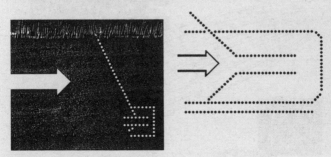

Bottle trap:

Cut a plastic bottle off just below the neck. Invert neck inside bottle. Use bait to entice them in. Once in, fish can't get out.

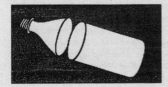 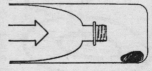

A similar trap can be made for larger fish using a hollow log. Make a lattice cone of twigs for the entrance and block the other end of the log.

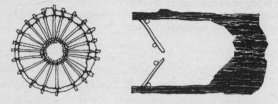

Wickerwork traps: Hazel or other pliant twigs can be used to make a trap which allows the current to flow through it and to a fish looks like stream-bottom debris.

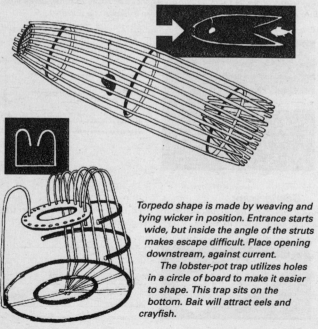

Torpedo shape is made by weaving and tying wicker in position. Entrance starts wide, but inside the angle of the struts makes escape difficult. Place opening downstream, against current.

The lobster-pot trap utilizes holes in a circle of board to make it easier to shape. This trap sits on the bottom. Bait will attract eels and crayfish.

OTHER TECHNIQUES

Fish snares: Large fish can be caught in a noose line fixed to the end of a pole, or passed down inside a length of bamboo. Pass loop over fish from tail end and pull up sharply so that the noose traps fish.

Eel bag: Tie fresh offal and straw or bracken in a cloth (not plastic) bag. Attach line and weight to end of bag and allow it to sink. Leave overnight and pull out in morning. Eels will chew their way into the bag and will still be wriggling in the straw when you land it.

Gill net: If you have a net, set floats at the top and weight the bottom, then stretch it across a river. It will soon empty a stretch of water, so do not use for long.

Attracting and driving: A torch held above water at night will draw fish. Draw nets to trap fish, then spear or club them. A mirror placed on the riverbed will reflect either sun or moonlight and attract fish.

Spearing: Sharpen a long stick to make a spear. Try to get above the fish and strike down swiftly. Make sure you are not casting a shadow over the fish. Aim slightly below it, to allow for the refraction of its image.

Muddying: Receding flood water leaves isolated pools. Stir up the mud at the bottom of the pool with a stick, or by stamping in the water. Fish will try to escape to clearer water. Scoop them out.

Explosives: Explosives kill nearby fish and force to the surface those which are farther away.

Guns: Fish can be shot in the water, but do not submerge the gun barrel—it will explode and the detonation will blow back at you.

Fish narcotics

Some plants stupefy fish to make them come to the surface. This works best in slack, warm waters. Do not use in closed pools—the fish supply can't be restocked.

> **The following plants are toxic only to cold-blooded animals, but should not be eaten by humans.**

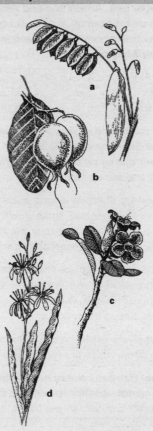

Derris (a) Occur SE Asia to Australia. Woody, vine-like plants with oval leaflets in opposite pairs, and purple flowers in seed pods. **Powder roots and throw them into the water.**

Barringtonia (b) Tree with same distribution as Derris, often near coasts. **Crush seeds inside their pods and throw into the water.**

Desert rose (Adenium) (c) Tropical and southern Africa, Arabia. Shrubs or small trees with thick fleshy leaves. The E. African species illustrated has spirals of blunt oval leaves and clusters of tubular pink flowers. **Crush stems and roots.**

Soap plant (d) N. America, dry open or scrubland. Narrow grass-like leaves, white star-like flowers. **Crush bulbous root and throw into the water.**

Dead fish floating on the surface—unless you have caused them to be there—may be diseased and unfit to eat.

ARCTIC FISHING

The technique of fishing through ice is effective on any frozen lake or river where the ice is thick enough to bear your weight but not so solid it can't be penetrated.

Bait the hook in the usual way. If line is carried back up against underside of ice, weight it below the hook. Set up multiple angling points. To signal when you have a bite, make a pennant from bright-colored cloth or card, and attach it to a light stick. Lash this firmly at right angles to another stick which extends the diameter of your hole by at least 30%. Now attach line to lower end of flagpole and rest flag on side of hole with line at its center. When fish takes bait, crosspiece will be pulled over hole and flag jerked upright. Be ready to pull your catch up quickly before a seal gets to it.

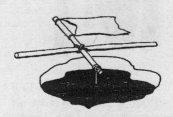 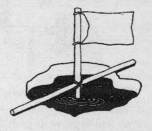

Ice netting: Make several holes in ice 40 cm (16 in) wide and twice that distance apart. Attach retaining loops to weighted net at intervals to match holes. Put loop at one end around a stick wider than the hole. With hooked pole, haul net through to next hole and anchor the next retaining loop. Continue until fully extended.

PREPARING FISH

All freshwater fish are edible. Those under 5 cm (2 in) long need no preparation: eat them whole. Larger fish must be gutted.

As soon as the fish is caught, cut its throat to bleed it, and remove gills. To gut it, slit from the anal orifice to the throat. Remove offal (use for hook bait). Keep roe, which runs down side of fish. Scaling is not necessary, but to scrape scales off draw knife from tail to head (a). Fish skin can be eaten. To skin eels and catfish, pass stake through fish, lodge it across two uprights, cut skin away and draw it down toward tail (b).

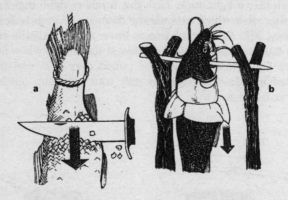

Preparing crustaceans: Eat as soon as possible. Boil for 20 minutes. Crabs have poisonous parts, so twist off claws and legs; with crab on its back, place your thumbs under flap at tail, push up. Pull flap up and away from body and lift off—this prevents stomach contents tainting flesh. Push down and out on mouth with your thumbs, to make mouth and stomach come away in one piece. Lungs are harmful: discard them.

CAMP CRAFT

I N a survival situation it is vital to know where to set up camp, how to build a shelter from the materials available, how to make fire, to cook and preserve food, and to improvise tools, clothing and equipment.

SHELTER AND MAKING CAMP

An accident, exhaustion, or sudden fog may leave you stranded. Local conditions and materials will determine the type of shelter you build. While there is still daylight to see by, scour the vicinity for the best natural shelter from wind, rain and cold before night sets in.

A wrecked plane or vehicle may provide shelter or materials from which one can be built, but if there is a risk of fire or fuel tanks exploding, wait until it has burned out before attempting salvage.

BAD PLACES TO CAMP

Exposed hilltops (go down, seek shelter on leeside).

Valley bottoms and deep hollows—damp and more liable to frost at night.

Hillside terraces where the ground holds moisture.

Spurs which lead down to water, which are often routes to animals' watering places.

Too close to water: you will be troubled by insects, and heavy rainfall may cause rivers to swell and flash floods to occur. Even old, dry watercourses are at risk.

Near solitary trees, which attract lightning.

Near bees' or hornets' nests.

WHERE TO CAMP

You should be sheltered from the wind, near water—but clear of any risk of flooding—with a plentiful supply of wood near at hand (in forest areas, keep to the edges where you can see and be seen). Check above your head for dead wood in trees that could crash down in a high wind. Don't camp across a game trail. Bear in mind that the sound of running water can drown out other noises which might indicate danger, or the sound of search parties.

TYPES OF SHELTER

For immediate protection, rig up a makeshift shelter while you construct something more permanent. If walking to safety, build temporary shelters at each halt; if sufficiently light, they can be carried with you.

Hasty shelters: Where no materials are available for constructing a shelter, make use of natural cover. In completely open plains, sit with your back to the wind and pile any equipment behind you as a windbreak.

Bough shelters: Branches that sweep down to the ground or partly broken boughs can provide shelter, but make sure they are not likely to fall off the tree.

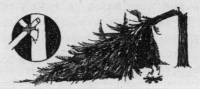

Make a similar shelter by lashing a broken-off bough to the base of another branch where it forks from the trunk (a).

Root shelter: The spreading roots and trapped earth at the base of a fallen tree make a good windbreak. Fill in the sides between extended roots for added shelter.

Natural hollows: Even a shallow depression will provide protection from the wind, but you must deflect any downhill flow of water if it is a hollow on a slope.

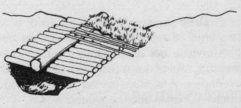

Make a roof to keep rain off and warmth in. A few sturdy branches laid across the hollow can support a light log laid over them, against which shorter sticks can be stacked to give pitch to the roof and so allow water to run off. Consolidate with turf, twigs and leaves.

Fallen trunks: A log makes a useful windbreak if it is at the right angle to the wind. With a small trunk, scoop out a hollow in the ground on the leeward side.

A log also makes an excellent support for a lean-to of boughs.

Drainage and ventilation: A run-off channel dug around any shelter in which you are below, or lying directly on, ground level will help keep you dry. Do not try to seal all gaps: ventilation is essential.

Stone barriers: A shelter is more comfortable if it is high enough to sit in, so increase its height by building a low wall of stones around your hollow. Caulk between the stones with turf and foliage mixed with mud.

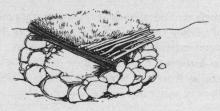

Sapling shelter: If suitable growth is available, select two lines of saplings, clear the ground between them of obstructions and lash the tops together to form a frame for sheeting. Weigh down the edges of the sheeting with rocks or timber. A similar shelter can be made from pliable branches driven into the ground.

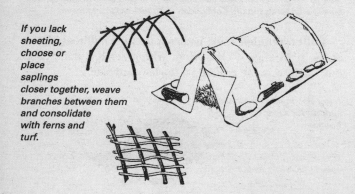

If you lack sheeting, choose or place saplings closer together, weave branches between them and consolidate with ferns and turf.

Shelter sheet: With a waterproof poncho, ground-sheet, plastic sheeting or canvas, a number of shelters can be made.

Make use of natural shelter (a) or make a triangular shelter with the apex pointing into the wind (b). Stake or weigh down edges. If it is long enough, curl the sheeting below you, running downhill (c). Use dry grass or bracken as bedding. Do not lie on cold or damp ground

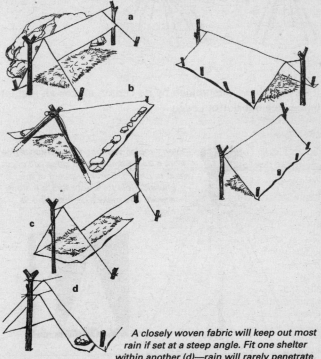

A closely woven fabric will keep out most rain if set at a steep angle. Fit one shelter within another (d)—rain will rarely penetrate both layers. Avoid touching the inner surface of woven fabric during rain—this draws water through.

Tepees: The quickest type to erect has three or more angled support poles, tied where they cross to make a cone. They can be tied on the ground and lifted into place before covering with hides, birch bark, or sheeting. Leave an opening at the top for ventilation.

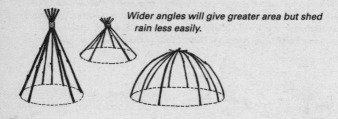

Wider angles will give greater area but shed rain less easily.

A parachute, suspended by its center, makes an instant tepee. Peg out bottom edge.

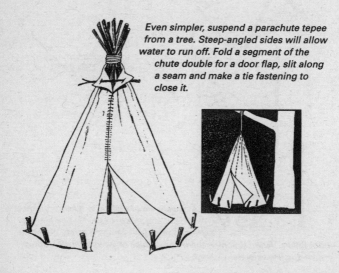

Even simpler, suspend a parachute tepee from a tree. Steep-angled sides will allow water to run off. Fold a segment of the chute double for a door flap, slit along a seam and make a tie fastening to close it.

Stick walls and screens

Build walls by piling sticks between uprights driven into the ground and (if possible) tied at the top. Use to make one side of a shelter, to block an opening, or for a heat reflector behind a fire. Can be used in place of large rocks to dam a stream.

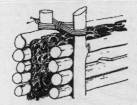

To make a very sturdy stick wall, increase the space between the uprights, use two stacks of sticks and fill the gap with earth.

Coverings: Use springy saplings, plant stems, grasses and long leaves to make wattle and woven coverings for roofs and walls. First make a framework from less pliable materials, either in situ or as a separate panel to attach later. Tie the main struts in position. Weave in the more pliant materials.

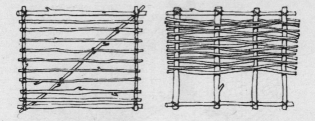

If no ties are available, drive vertical stakes into the ground and weave saplings between them. Caulk with earth and grasses.

If suitable firm crosspieces are scarce, weave creepers between the uprights. Very large leaves, lashed or weighted down, can be overlapped like tiles or shingles to keep out rain.

Long grass can be bunched and woven, or use birch bark to make tiles. Ring a birch tree with even 60 cm (2 ft) cuts and remove bark (a). Fix pairs of canes or creepers across a frame (b). Upper ends of tiles are gripped between the canes; lower ends rest on those below (c).

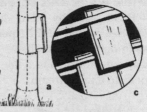

Open lean-to shelter: If there is nothing to lean a roof against (and no need to keep out heavy rain or blizzards) use panels of wattle or grass-covered frames.

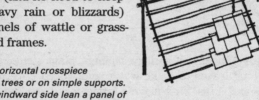

Erect a horizontal crosspiece between trees or on simple supports. On the windward side lean a panel of wattle, or lean saplings at 45° to make a roof. Add side walls (a). Site your fire on the leeward and build a reflector (b) on the other side to prevent heat escaping.

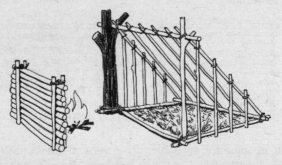

Tropical shelters

In rain forests and jungle where the ground is damp and crawling with insects a raised bed is preferable. Unless the nights are cold, the number one priority will be to keep reasonably dry. The following are useful materials.

Bamboo: A very versatile building material found in damp places from India through to China, parts of Africa, Australia and the southern USA and which can be used for supports, flooring, roofing and walls.

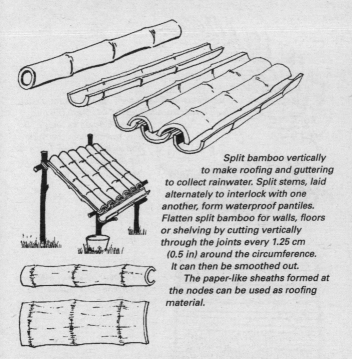

Split bamboo vertically to make roofing and guttering to collect rainwater. Split stems, laid alternately to interlock with one another, form waterproof pantiles. Flatten split bamboo for walls, floors or shelving by cutting vertically through the joints every 1.25 cm (0.5 in) around the circumference. It can then be smoothed out.

The paper-like sheaths formed at the nodes can be used as roofing material.

Take great care when collecting bamboo. Some stems are under tension and when cut explode into sharp slivers. Split bamboo can be razor-sharp and cause serious injury. The husks at the base of bamboo stems carry small stinging hairs which cause severe skin irritations.

Thatch of leaves: Atap and other large leaves when thatched make the best roofs and walls for jungle shelters. Look for any plant similarly structured, the bigger and broader the better.

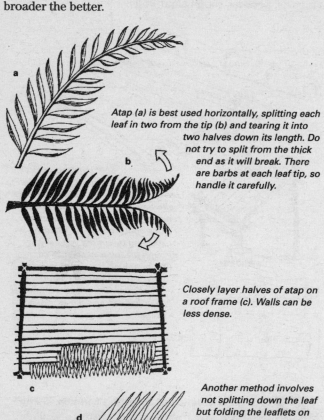

Atap (a) is best used horizontally, splitting each leaf in two from the tip (b) and tearing it into two halves down its length. Do not try to split from the thick end as it will break. There are barbs at each leaf tip, so handle it carefully.

Closely layer halves of atap on a roof frame (c). Walls can be less dense.

Another method involves not splitting down the leaf but folding the leaflets on one side across to the other and interweaving them (d). This is easiest if you work from one side then the other, but requires practice.

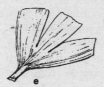 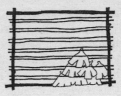

Three-lobed leaves or leaves cut in this fashion (e) can be locked over a thatching frame without any other fixing being necessary to hold them in place (f).

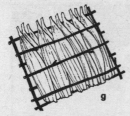 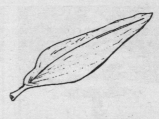

Elephant grass and other large leaves can be woven between the cross-pieces (g). Only a small number are needed to produce a shelter very quickly.

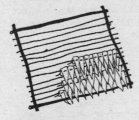 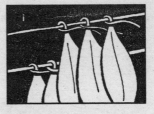

Long broad leaves can be sown along the thatching battens with vines (h).

Palm and other long-stemmed leaves can be secured by carrying the stem around the batten and over the front of the leaf, where it is held by the next leaf (i). Leaves must overlap those below on the outside of the shelter.

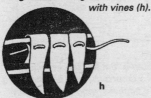

Arctic shelters

In polar areas caves and hollows form simple shelters. If you carry a bivouac, increase its protection by piling up loose snow around and over it, so long as it can support the weight. At very low temperatures snow is solid and you need spades and ice saws to cut into it or make blocks of it.

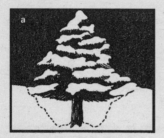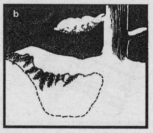

Snow or rock caves are easily recognizable, but look also for spaces left beneath conifers when snow has built up around them. A medium-sized tree may have a space right around the trunk (a) or large one may have pockets in the snow beneath a branch (b). Try digging under any tree with spreading branches on the lee side.

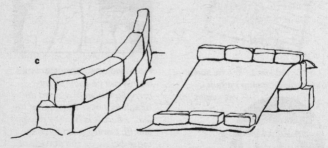

Even soft snow can be built into a windbreak. Cut and stack blocks (c). Use another course of blocks to anchor a ground sheet or poncho along the top, use others to secure the bottom edge and more to close the sides.

BUILDING IN SNOW
Cut compacted snow—using a saw, knife, shovel or machete—into blocks 45 x 50 cm (18 x 20 in) and 10–20 cm (4–8 in) thick. These will provide good insulation while allowing the sun's rays to penetrate.

Snow trench: This is a one-person shelter for short-term use only. Mark out an area the size of a sleeping bag; cut out blocks the whole width of the trench. Dig down at least 60 cm (2 ft). Along the top of the sides cut a ledge c. 15 cm (6 in) wide and the same depth.

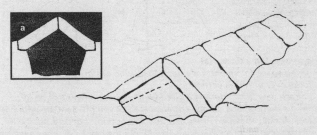

Rest snow bricks on each side of the ledge and lean them in against each other to form a roof (a).

Put equipment under sleeping bag as insulation. Block windward end with a block or piled snow. At the downwind end, dig an entrance, or have a removable block as a door. Fill gaps with snow. This shelter is best built on a slight slope with entrance at lower end.

Snow cave: Dig into a drift of firm snow. Create three levels inside: build a fire on the highest, sleep on the center one and keep off the lower level which will trap the cold. Drive two holes through the roof: one for a chimney and one to ensure adequate ventilation.

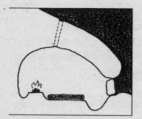

Use a block of snow as a door, keeping it loose fitting and on the inside so it won't jam. Smooth inside surfaces to discourage drips, and make a channel around the internal perimeter for melt.

Igloo: An efficient snow house. Make sure entrance does not face into wind (erect windbreak if necessary).

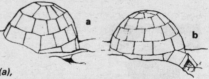

Mark out a circle 4 m (13.5 ft) in diameter and tramp it down to consolidate the floor. Cut and lay circle of blocks on perimeter. Dig a tunnel (a), leaving space for an entrance (b). Add a layer, centering new blocks over previous vertical joint.

Each new layer should be placed halfway over lower tier, so igloo forms a dome shape. Shape entrance arch as you go. Seal top with flat block. Make ventilation holes near top and bottom (not on side of prevailing wind, or so low that snow blocks the hole). Fill other gaps with snow. Smooth off the inside to remove drip-points.

Inside the igloo, build a sleeping level higher than the floor and create a lower cold level for storage.

Sweating is to be avoided, so take your time over building a complex structure and rest frequently.

Adequate ventilation is essential to prevent carbon monoxide poisoning and to allow moisture to escape.

The smaller the shelter, the warmer it will be, but it will not be possible to heat it much above freezing.

LIVING IN A SNOW HOUSE

Make sure you have a supply of fuel in the shelter.

Knock snow off boots and clothing before entering.

Mark the entrance so that it is easily found.

Keep shovels and tools inside to dig yourself out.

Stop drips by placing a piece of snow on the source.

Relieve yourself indoors in containers.

No matter how low the external temperature, that inside a snow house will not drop below -10°C (0°F). An oil burner or fat on bones are alternative heating fuels when there is no wood or casiope.

Long-term shelters

If you decide that there is no hope of rescue and it is impracticable to make your own way to safety due to distance, time of year, lack of equipment or physical condition, make a comfortable, permanent shelter.

Caves: Those situated above a valley will be dry even if water seeps through in some places from above. They are weather-proof and require little aside from a barrier of rocks or wattle to close off the entrance. Caves may be inhabited by wild animals, so approach with caution. Dry plant matter on the ground will provide insulation. A good fire will make animals leave (allow them an escape route). Build the fire at the back of the cave so smoke goes up to the roof—smoke from a fire near the open mouth of a cave will be blown in. If you seal the entrance, make sure to leave a gap for smoke to escape.

Check for the possibility of a rock fall inside or outside the cave. You could be trapped or injured by falling rocks.

Light structures: Follow the methods outlined for the lean-to structure (p. 110). Extend it with a less angled roof and a front wall, or build vertical walls and roof them over with deep eaves to give extra shade and to ensure that rain runs off. In hot climates the walls can then be fairly open lattice to allow air to pass through. Grasses and mud will seal cracks. In climates with heavy rainfall, use leaves or bark-like tiles on top.

If you have bamboo or other strong material to build a firm frame in tropical climates, raise the floor of your shelter off the ground to keep out other creatures.

Sod house: Cut sections of turf 45 x 15 cm (18 x 6 in) and build with them like bricks, overlapping them to form a bond. Keep the structure low—big enough to sit but not to stand in. One side could be open, facing your fire. Slope the sides to give pitch to the roof, which will be supported by spars of wood. Lay turves on the roof as well, or cover it with grass.

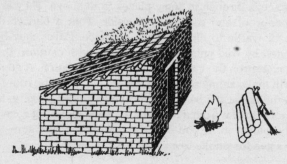

FIRE

Fire is essential to survival. It provides warmth, protection and a means of signaling; it boils water, cooks and preserves food; it heats metal to make tools and bake pots. You must learn to light a fire anywhere under any conditions. It is not enough to know all the methods—you have to be expert at them.

 Remember the Fire Triangle.
Its three sides represent air, heat, and fuel.
If any one of these is removed, the triangle collapses and the fire goes out.

PREPARATION

Ensure adequate ventilation for your fire. The more oxygen introduced, the brighter the fire; by reducing ventilation the fire burns less fiercely, needing less fuel. Collect sufficient supplies of tinder, kindling and fuel. Prepare a fireplace so you can control the fire.

The fireplace

Choose a sheltered site. Except for signal purposes (see pp. 211–213), do not light a fire at the base of a tree. Clear away leaves, twigs, moss and dry grass from a circle 2 m (6 ft) across until you have a bare earth surface.

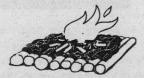 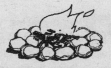

If the ground is wet or snow-covered, build a platform from a layer of green logs covered with a layer of earth, or a layer of stones.

Temple fire:

A raised platform of green timber. Four uprights support crosspieces in their forks. Place a layer of green logs across them and cover this with several inches of earth. Light the fire on top of this. A pole across upper forks on diagonally opposite uprights can support cooking pots.

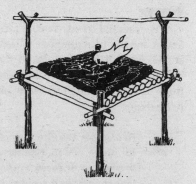

In windy conditions dig a trench and light your fire in it.

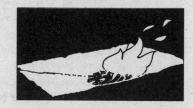

Alternatively, encircle your fire with rocks to retain heat and save fuel. They serve as heated potstands and can be used as bedwarmers.

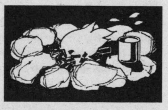

Avoid placing wet or porous rocks near fires, especially rocks which have been submerged in water—they may explode when heated, producing dangerous flying fragments which could take out an eye if you are close to the fire. Avoid slates and softer rocks. Test them by banging them together, and do not use any that crack or sound hollow.

Tinder

Tinder is any material that takes only a spark to ignite. Birch bark, dried grasses, wood shavings, bird down, waxed paper, cotton fluff, fir cones, pine needles, powdered dried fungi, scorched or charred cotton are excellent tinder, as is the fine dust produced by wood-burrowing insects and the inside of birds' nests.

Kindling

Kindling is the wood used to raise flames from tinder. Small dry twigs, resinous and softer woods are best.

Tinder and kindling must be dry. Don't collect it from the earth. If the outside of kindling is damp, shave until you reach dry wood.

Make fire sticks
Shave sticks with shallow cuts to "feather" them. This will make the wood catch light more quickly.

Fuel

Use dry wood to get a fire going. Once established, mix green and dried-out damp wood.

Hard woods such as hickory, beech and oak, burn well, are long lasting, and give off great heat.

Soft woods burn fast and give off sparks: the worst culprits are alder, spruce, pine, chestnut and willow.

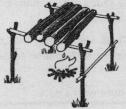

Dry wood across two supports high enough above a fire that they won't be set alight. Lay green logs beside fire, tapering away from the wind, so they shelter the fire while they dry.

A basic woodshed is vital in wet weather. Position where fire will warm it, but clear of stray sparks.

Save energy: don't chop logs, break them over a rock (a).

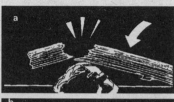

Or feed them over the fire, letting them burn through in the middle (b).

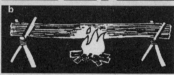

Split logs without an axe by placing a knife on the end of a log and hitting it with a rock (c). Once begun, split can be widened with wooden wedge plugged in gap and driven downward. Don't do this if you have only one knife—it could get damaged.

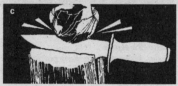

OTHER FUELS

Animal droppings: dry well, mix with grass and leaves.

Peat: found on moors. Soft and springy underfoot, it looks black and fibrous. Dry it before burning. Needs ventilation when burning.

Coal: sometimes found on surface in northern tundra.

Shales: rich in oil, burn readily. Some sands also contain oil and burn with a thick smoke—good signals.

Combustibles: petroleum, hydraulic fluid, engine oils, insect repellent. Soaked in oil, tires, upholstery and rubber seals are inflammable.

Animal fats: use a tin for a stove and burn with a wick.

Burning oil and water:

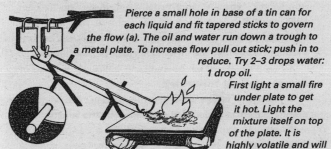

Pierce a small hole in base of a tin can for each liquid and fit tapered sticks to govern the flow (a). The oil and water run down a trough to a metal plate. To increase flow pull out stick; push in to reduce. Try 2–3 drops water: 1 drop oil.

First light a small fire under plate to get it hot. Light the mixture itself on top of the plate. It is highly volatile and will burn almost anything.

Burning oils:

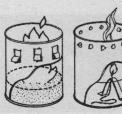

Mix gasoline with sand and burn in ventilated tin, or dig fire pit. Burn oil by mixing in gasoline or antifreeze. Do not set a light directly to any liquid fuels: make a wick for flame.

FIRELIGHTING

Form a tepee of kindling around tinder bed. If windy, lean kindling against a log on the leeside. Ignite tinder. Add larger sticks once kindling has caught. Or light a bundle of dry match-thin twigs and place in tepee.

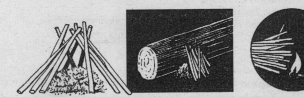

Matches are the easiest way to start a fire. Carry the non-safety type in waterproof containers, packed so they can't rub, rattle or ignite. Split in half to make them go further. To strike split matches, press inflammable end against the striking surface with a finger.

Strike a damp match by stabbing obliquely instead of drawing it along striker strip.

If your hair is dry and not too greasy, roll a damp match in it. Static electricity will dry out the match.

Whenever you strike a match, light a candle. Many things can then be lit from it, saving matches. Even a small candle will last a long time if used carefully.

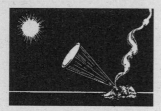

Sunlight through a lens: *can ignite tinder. Use your survival kit magnifying glass, telescope or camera lens. Focus sun's rays to form a tiny, bright spot of light. Keep it steady and shield from wind. Blow it gently as it glows.*

Powder from ammunition: *Break open a round and pour gunpowder on tinder (a) and use flint. Or leave half the powder in cartridge case and stuff piece of cloth in (b). Chamber the round and fire into the ground. The smoldering cloth will be ejected. Place on tinder to ignite.*

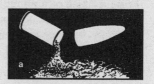
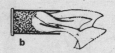

Flint: A stone found in many parts of the world. Strike with steel and hot sparks fly off (a). Or use saw-edged blade from survival kit (b) for more sparks.

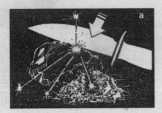
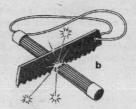

Battery firelighting: Attach two lengths of wire to battery. If you have no wire, use metal tools. If using a car battery, remove it from the vehicle first.

Slowly bring bare ends of two pieces of wire together. A spark will jump across just before they touch. Aim it at tinder. A small piece of cloth with a little petrol is best tinder for this.

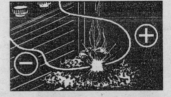

Fire bow: The friction of a hardwood spindle rotated on a softwood base produces wood-dust tinder, then heat. Both spindle and base must be dry.

Gouge a small depression at near end of baseboard. Cut a cavity below for tinder. Shape the spindle evenly. Make a bow from a pliable shoot and hide, twine or a bootlace. Use hollow piece of stone/wood to steady top of the spindle and exert downward pressure. Wind bowstring once around spindle. Place spindle in the depression, hold steadying piece over its end and bear down lightly while moving bow backward and forward so spindle spins. Increase speed as spindle starts drilling. When it enters cavity, apply more pressure and bow vigorously.

Keep spindle upright and steady, and bow strokes even. It helps to kneel with one foot on baseboard. Carry on bowing until a glowing tip drops on to tinder. Blow on it gently to ignite.

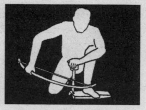

Hand drill: A variation on the fire bow.

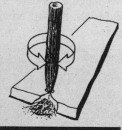

Cut a V-shaped notch in hardwood baseboard. Make a small depression. Use stem of hollow softwood with soft pith core for spindle. Roll the spindle between the palms of your hands, running hands down it as you go to press it into depression.

When friction makes the spindle tip glow red, blow gently to ignite the tinder. Put a pinch of sand in spindle hole to increase friction.

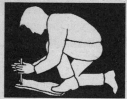

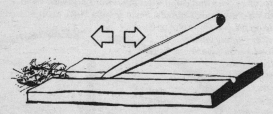

Fire plough:

Cut a straight groove in a softwood baseboard and then plough the tip of a hardwood shaft up and down it. This produces tinder, then ignites it.

FIRELIGHTING WITH CHEMICALS

The following mixtures can be ignited by grinding with rocks or putting them under friction point in a fire drill. Mix carefully and avoid contact with metal. Keep dry.

Potassium chlorate and sugar in a 3:1 mix.
Potassium permanganate and sugar mixed 9:1.
Sodium chlorate and sugar mixed 3:1.

Potassium chlorate is found in some throat tablets.
Potassium permanganate is part of your survival kit.
Sodium chlorate is a weed-killer.

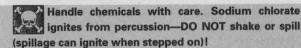

Handle chemicals with care. Sodium chlorate ignites from percussion—DO NOT shake or spill (spillage can ignite when stepped on)!

TYPES OF FIRE

Fires for warmth

Only surfaces facing an outdoor fire are warmed by it.

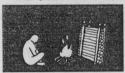

A reflector not only reflects heat but makes smoke go upward. Use one to reflect heat into a sleeping shelter.

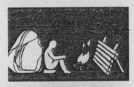

Site fire near a rock. Sit between the two so that the rock reflects the heat and warms your back. Add a reflector.

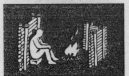

If there is no rock to reflect heat, build a second reflector to go behind you.

Snake hole fire: In the side of a firm earth bank dig a chamber about 45 cm (18 in) deep. From above, drive a stick down into the chamber, maneuver it a little to make a chimney, removing the spoil that falls below.

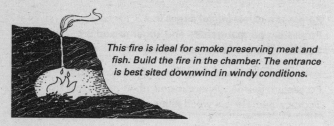

This fire is ideal for smoke preserving meat and fish. Build the fire in the chamber. The entrance is best sited downwind in windy conditions.

Cooking fires
Trench fire:

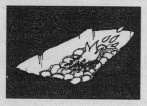

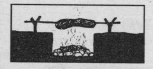

Dig a trench 30 x 90cm (12 x 36 in) and 30 cm (12 in) deep plus the depth of a layer of rocks with which you now line the bottom. Build a fire on the rocks. Even when it dies down, they will remain hot enough to make a grill. A spit placed across the embers is ideal for roasts.

Hobo stove:

Punch holes in the bottom and around the bottom sides of a 5-gallon oil drum. Cut out a panel on one side, 5 cm (2 in) from the bottom, through which to stoke the fire. Set the drum on a ring of stones to allow ventilation beneath.

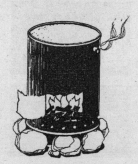

COOKING

Cooking makes food more appetizing and easy to digest. It destroys bacteria and parasites that may be present, and neutralizes poisons. But when heated, food loses nutritional value. Never cook longer than necessary.

Use the fire to boil water, then let the flames die down and use embers and hot ash for cooking.

Never leave your fire unattended when cooking.

Having lit a fire, always have water boiling—unless in short supply—for drinks, sterilizing wounds, etc.

Do not just balance a can on the fire. Support vessels on rocks or suspend them over the fire, for stability.

COOKING METHODS

Boiling: Cans and metal boxes are ideal for boiling water. Make a handle, hang them from a pot support or use tongs to move them. Punctures can be repaired by hammering in small plugs of wood—when wet they will expand and stop leaks. Improvise pots from a thick length of bamboo or sections of birch bark—but do not let them boil dry.

To cook in a bamboo stem, angle it across the heat of the fire, supporting it on a forked stick driven into the ground.

Boiling conserves natural juices—always drink the liquid unless boiling out toxic substances.

Any dead animal that is not actually decomposing can be eaten if you use only the large muscle areas. Cut into 2.5 cm (1 in) cubes and boil for 30 mins. Eat only a little, and wait half-hour—most toxins act in that time or less. If there are no ill effects, dig in.

Roasting: Skewer the meat on a spit and turn it over hot embers or beside a blazing fire. Continually turn meat to keep the fat moving over the surface.

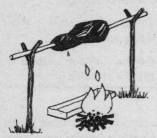

A spit should be set to one side of fire to allow for a drip tray to catch fat for basting. Fierce heat cooks the outside, leaving the inside undercooked, so a slow roast is best. Cut off outer meat, then continue roasting to cook the inner flesh.

Grilling: Wastes fat—use only when food is plentiful.

Rest a wire mesh or a grid of green sticks on rocks over the embers. Or use a long stick on a forked support to hold food over the fire. Wrap the food around the stick.

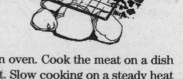

Baking: This requires an oven. Cook the meat on a dish and baste it with its own fat. Slow cooking on a steady heat tenderizes meat. Baking is also ideal for root vegetables.

A large metal box with a hinged lid and a catch you can use as a handle, can be set up to open sideways. If it has no catch let it open downward. Place a support in front, to rest lid on. Prop it closed and avoid a tight fit which could build up dangerous pressure inside. If no box is available, make a clay dome, set a fire inside and scrape this out before cooking. Leave a small aperture which can be easily sealed while baking.

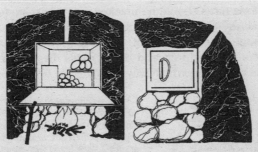

Stand the box on rocks so a fire can be lit under it. Build up rocks and earth or clay around the back, sides and top, but leave a space behind and make a chimney hole from above leading to this space.

Steaming: Is a good way to cook fish and vegetables. Punch holes in a can and suspend it inside a larger can, or put something in the bottom of the large can to keep the inner one above water. Cover the outer can, but do not seal it or the pressure could cause it to explode.

Improvise a steamer of bamboo: between the inner compartments make a hole just big enough to let water through to fill the bottom section. Make a lid (not too tight) for the top. Water boiled in the lowest section will produce steam to cook food in the top one.

Frying: A good way to vary diet, if fat is available. Any sheet of metal that can be fashioned into a curve will serve to fry in. Some large leaves (e.g., banana) contain enough oil not to dry out before the cooking is done. Try the leaves out first before cooking food on them and fry only over embers.

Cooking in clay: This requires no utensils. Wrap food in a ball of clay and place in the embers. Heat radiates through the clay, which protects against food scorching.

Animals must be cleaned and gutted first but need not be otherwise prepared: when the clay is removed spines, scales or feathers from small birds come away with it, but big birds should be plucked. Not advisable for root vegetables—skins are too nutritious to lose.

Hangi: Another way of cooking without utensils. It requires kindling, logs and round rocks the size of a fist. Do not use stones which may explode (see p. 120).

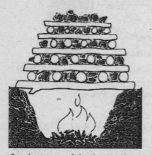

Dig an oval hole with rounded sides 45–60 cm deep (18–24 in); place kindling at the bottom. Lay logs across the hole, place another layer at right angles, interspersed with stones. Build up 5 or 6 more alternating layers, and top off with stones.

When the kindling is set alight the logs will burn, heating the stones above them, until, eventually, all falls into the pit.

Remove embers and ash, place food on top of the hot rocks, meat in center and vegetables to the edge. There must be a gap between the food and earth. Lay saplings across the pit and cover with sacking, leaves and earth. Uncover after 1½ hours; your meal is ready.

The hangi can be used to boil water collected in a waterproof sack, provided the fabric won't melt. Place tied-up sack in the hangi. Takes about 1½ hours to boil.

Useful Utensils

Tongs:
Lash 2 branches so they spring apart at the ends—use a tapering piece of wood between them under the lashings. Grip is improved if one has forked end. Use for holding hot pots.

Pot rod:

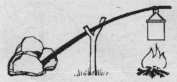

Drive a sturdy forked stick into ground near fire. Rest a longer stick across it with one end over fire. Drive bottom of long stick in ground and weight with rocks. Cut a groove near the tip to prevent pots slipping off, or tie on a strong hook.

Swinging pot holder:

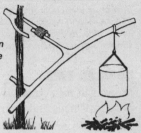

Bind 2 forked sticks together so forks fit in opposite directions on a firm upright. The cantilever action will maintain the height you set it at, and a push sideways will swing the pot away from the flames.

Variable pot hook:

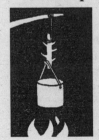

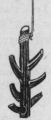

Cut a strong piece with several branches from a small tree or bush and trim branches to 10–12 cm (4–5 in). Strip off the bark, which may hide rotten wood.

Cup:

Cut a section of bamboo just below a joint, then cut just below the next joint up. Smooth the edges to prevent splinters.

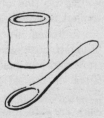

Spoon:

Scribe a spoon shape on a flattish piece of wood with a knife point. Whittle to required shape. Never cut toward yourself.

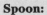

Birch bark containers:

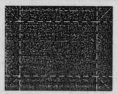
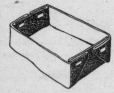

*Use the inner layer of bark to make cooking vessels.
Sew or tie them near the top to prevent unfolding.
Make a second vessel with a larger base for a lid.*

*A circle, folded into quarters, will make a cone-
shaped cup or a boiling vessel if suspended.*

COOKING TIPS

Meat: Cut into cubes and boil. Venison is prone to worms,
pork to worms and liver fluke. Marinate tough meat in citric juice for 24 hours before cooking.

Offal: Check liver: only if firm, odorless, free from spots
and hard lumps can it be eaten. Boil, then fry if you wish.
Hearts: par-boil then bake. Brains: skin head and boil, sim-
mering for 90 minutes. Strip all flesh from the skull, including the eyes, tongue and ears. Blood: collect in a container
and leave covered until a clear liquid comes to the top. When
separation seems complete drain it off. Dry the residue by
the fire to form a firm cake. Use to enrich soups and stews.

Fish: Stew or wrap in leaves and place in hot embers
(avoid toxic leaves).

Birds: Boil all carrion. Old birds are tough and best
boiled. Stuff young ones with herbs or fruits and then roast.

Reptiles: Gut, then cook in their skins. Place in hot
embers, turning continually. When skin splits meat can be
removed and boiled. Some snakes have poisonous secre-
tions on the skin and others have venom glands in their
head, so cut this off before cooking. If you are not sure
they are safe, take care in handling them. Skin frogs (many
have poisonous skins) then roast on a stick.

Shark: Cut into small cubes and soak overnight in fresh water. Boil in several changes of water to get rid of the ammonia flavor.

Shellfish: Safest boiled. All seafood spoils quickly. Drop into boiling salted water and boil for 10 minutes.

Insects and worms: Best boiled. Cook and mince them by crushing in a can. Or dry on hot rocks, then grind into a powder with which to enrich soups and stews.

Eggs: Boil, or roast after first using a sharp stick or knifepoint to pierce a small hole in one end. Place on warm embers to cook slowly. If a boiled egg contains an embryo chick remove the embryo and roast it.

Green vegetables: Wash and boil until tender. Can be steamed if you are sure they are safe. Add to stew after the meat is cooked. Eat fresh greens raw as salad.

Roots: Any toxins are destroyed by heat. Try boiling for 5 minutes, then place in a hole dug beneath the fire, cover with ash and embers and leave until tender.

Lichens and mosses: Soak overnight. Add to stews.

Sago: Fell a sago palm at base of the trunk and trim the tip just below last flowering line. Divide the trunk into sections cut lengthwise. Using each section as a trough, pound pith into a mash, then knead in a container of water and strain through a cloth. A starchy paste will form in the water. Roll this into sticky balls and cook.

Palm sap: Choose a fat stalk carrying a flowering head (at the base of the crown on trunk). Bruise with a club, then cut off head. Sweet juice will flow from end of stalk. Bruise and cut daily to stimulate flow. Drink raw or boil, then cool to produce lumps of pure sugar.

PRESERVING FOOD

If food is not plentiful or is limited by season, ensure that stores keep safely.

Do not store food in direct sunlight, near excessive warmth or moisture, nor where scavengers may ruin it.

Wrap in airtight and waterproof materials—or store in containers with a good seal. Label stores and separate different foods to avoid cross-flavoring.

Check occasionally to see all is well.

DRYING

Wind and sun can dry food but it is easier to force-dry over a fire. Dried foods are less vulnerable to molds and maggots. Meat with a high fat content is difficult to preserve. Cut off most of the fat and rub salt into the flesh. Hang the salted meat in a cool airy place.

Smoking: This dehydrates meat and coats it with a protective layer. Smoking can be carried out in a smoke tepee. Get a fire going to produce hot embers. Have a pile of green leaves ready.

To build a smoke tepee, drive three sticks into the ground to form a triangle and tie the tops together. Build a platform between them and set a fire beneath.

Hardwood leaves are ideal, but avoid holly and other toxic leaves, and conifers which may burst into flame. Do not use grass. Make sure there are no flames left, and pile leaves over the embers.

Cut meat into fat-free strips, 2.5 cm (1 in) by 6 mm (½ in), gut and fillet fish. Cover the tepee with a cloth to keep in the smoke. If you don't have a cloth, pile boughs and turfs on the frame and seal it. Leave for 18 hours and ensure little or no smoke escapes.

To avoid risk of embers setting tepee alight, build a snake hole fire (see p. 128); erect tepee over chimney.

Biltong: Cut strips, as for smoking; hang them in sun, out of reach of animals, 2–3 m (6–10 ft) above ground. They can take 2 weeks to dry. Protect them from rain and dew. Turn the strips to ensure all surfaces are dried, and keep flies off so they don't lay eggs.

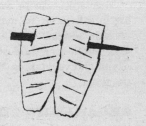

To dry fish, cut off the head, tail and gut. Split open, remove the backbone and score inner flesh. Lay on hot, sun-baked rocks. Fish less than 7.5 cm (3 in) long need not be gutted.

Fish can also be smoked. They will be easier to hang if cleaned and gutted without removing the backbone, head or tail. Suspend by one side of the head.

Pemmican: This is concentrated food made from biltong, ideal for provisions to carry on treks. Before setting out, take equal quantities, by weight, of biltong and rendered fat. Shred and pound the meat. Melt the animal fat over the shredded meat and mix together well. When cold pack in a waterproof bag. It will keep for a long time, especially in cold climates.

Nuts and cereals

Place on hot rocks from the fire, turning frequently until dried. Store in damp-proof containers.

Fruit, fungi and lichens

Fruit and berries can be dried whole or cut into slices and dried by sun, smoke or heat. Fungi also dry easily. Fruit can be eaten dry. Add fungi to soups or soak in water for several hours to regain their texture.

To store lichens, soak overnight, boil well and allow to dry. Grind to a powder, then boil again to form a thick syrup, which adds body to other foods.

PICKLING AND SALTING

Citric acid from limes and lemons can be used to pickle fish and meat. Dilute juice and water 2:1, mix well and soak the flesh for at least 12 hours. Transfer it to an airtight container with enough solution to cover meat.

Vegetables can be preserved by boiling and then keeping in saltwater. To make sure a brine solution is strong enough, add salt until a potato or root vegetable will float in it. Another method of using salt is to tightly pack layers of salt and vegetables. Wash off the salt when you need to use them.

ORGANIZING THE CAMP

If no command structure exists between a group of survivors, establish an organizing committee with particular responsibilities. A roster is essential for daily chores. Everyone who is fit should take their turn at unpleasant tasks, unless their skills are in such demand that it would be a waste of their abilities.

Keeping busy eliminates boredom and keeps up morale. Invalids should get light jobs. At all times there must be someone in camp able to operate the signals should a search aircraft appear. If numbers permit, avoid venturing from the camp in less than pairs.

A nightly gathering will provide discipline, and an opportunity to debrief and to discuss new strategies.

Boredom is dangerous for a lone survivor and objectives should be set each day whether practical or for amusement. A regular routine helps morale.

CAMP HYGIENE

Strict hygiene should be practiced in the camp.

CAMP LAYOUT

Latrines must be downhill of camp and away from the water supply to avoid risk of seepage.

Establish a collection point for drinking water. Ensure no one washes upstream of it. Downstream choose a point for ablutions and laundry, and downstream of that a place for cleaning cooking utensils.

Latrines and rubbish disposal should be well away from camp—preferably downwind—but not so far as to be inconvenient. Cut a track to make access easier.

Never urinate or defecate near your water supply. Latrines must be established, even for a lone survivor. Do not use disinfectant—after defecating cover feces with earth. Make a latrine cover to keep out flies and always replace it. If a latrine starts to smell, dig a new one. Fill in the old latrine and burn old timbers.

Deep trench latrine:

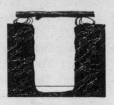

Dig a trench 1.25 m (4 ft) deep and 45 cm (18 in) wide. Build up sides with logs, rocks or earth to sitting height. Seal gaps. Lay logs across to leave only a hole for use. Pour wood ash on logs to make a seal and deter flies.

Cover opening with wooden lid, flat rock or a large leaf weighted with stones.

Urinal:

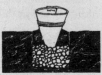

Dig a pit 60 cm (2 ft) deep. Fill it three-quarters full with large stones and top up with earth, with a bark cone set into it as a funnel.

Incinerator: Rubbish should be burned. Make a fire in the latrine area using a large can as an incinerator. Bury unburned refuse in a pit.

CAMP DISCIPLINE

Do not prepare game in camp: bleed, gut and skin on the trap line to attract game to traps, not to the camp.

Keep food covered and off the ground.

Replace lids on containers immediately after use.

Stow clothing and equipment where it cannot get wet or burned. Keep things tidy: hook mess tins and cooking utensils on twigs and branches.

Never leave the fire unattended.

Soap: Washing with soap leaves skin less waterproof and more prone to attack by germs. However, soap is an antiseptic, better than many others, such as iodine, which destroy body tissue as well as germs. It is ideal for scrubbing hands before administering first-aid. Save supplies for this.

Soap-making: Two ingredients—an oil and alkali—are needed. The oil can be animal fat or vegetable, but not mineral. The alkali can be produced by burning wood or seaweed to produce ash.

To make soap, wash the ash with water, then strain and boil it with the oil. Simmer until excess liquid is evaporated and allow to cool. This soap is not antiseptic. Add horseradish root or pine resin to make it antiseptic. Too much alkali in the mix will dry the skin, leaving it sore.

TOOLS

Stone tools: Split a cobble with a blow from a hard, smooth pebble to form a flat face. The blow should be at an angle of less than 90°. Shape by hitting edge-on with another stone (a), then create a platform on one side (b) from which a series of flakes can be struck vertically down (c). Then strike with softer stones, and hit and press small flakes away with a piece of antler or hard wood. Flakes may be used as scrapers, to cut edges, and as arrowheads.

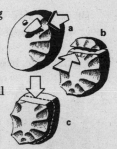

Bone tools: Bones, antlers and horns make useful digging implements, gougers and hammers. Cut them with stone tools or grind with coarse stones. A shoulder blade is a good shape for a saw (a). First split in half, then teeth can be cut along it with a knife. A small bone scraper (b) could also be made, the edge ground sharp. Ribs are ideal for shaping into points (c).

To make a bone needle, choose a suitably sized bone and sharpen to a point. Burn an eye with a piece of hot wire, or scrape with a knife point or piece of flint. Don't heat the knife in the fire.

AXES

To improvise a handle for an axe-head use any straight, knot-free hardwood. The flukes of a buttress tree (a) are ideal; slightly curved, straight-grained and easy to work. Cut two notches into the fluke of a buttress, spaced to the desired length (b to c).

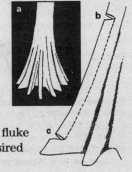

Hit along side of fluke close to the cuts. It will split away at their depth.

Fitting the head: Whittle the handle into shape with one end cut to fit the hole in the axehead, cutting a notch in that end. Make a wedge to fit the notch. With the head in place drive in the notch, then soak the axe in water overnight to tighten head on the shaft. Always check axeheads for tightness before using.

   To fit a stone axehead: Select a hardwood handle. Tie a band of cord around it 23 cm (9 in) from one end. Split end as far as this band (use a knife and a wedge or the axehead flint). Insert flint and tie end.

Sharpening an axe: Use a file to get rid of burrs, and a whetstone to impart the sharp edge. A file is a one-way tool—it works when pushed, not pulled.

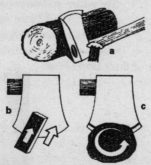

Prop axehead between a log and a peg (a). Always sharpen inward from cutting edge to avoid producing burrs.

   Use file or rougher stone first to remove and burrs (b). Finish with a smooth stone, using a circular motion. Don't drag stone off cutting edge. Push on to blade. (See pp. 11–14.)

   Turn axe over. Repeat process circling in opposite direction (c).

Using an axe: Swing an axe in an arc that feels natural with a firm grip and always away from your body, hands, and legs. Make sure that, if you miss your target and follow through the axe will not strike you or anyone else. Never throw an axe on the ground. Sheath it or bury the blade in a log.

Tree felling

Check overhead for dead branches and hornets' nests. Clear creepers and branches which could deflect blows. Cut branches off from the outside of the join.

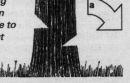

Cut from both sides of the tree, first chopping out a notch at an angle of 45° and another on the opposite side at a lower level, on the side to which you want the tree to fall (a). Do not cut more than halfway before starting the other notch.

A tree with most of its branches on one side will fall in that direction regardless of the placing of the cuts.

Use a steady rhythm of blows. Put too much effort behind the axe and your aim will suffer. Alternating the angle of stroke will prevent the axe from jamming. Too steep an angle will cause the axe to glance off, dead-on will make it jam or be inefficient. Aim for 45°.

Splitting logs:
Stand behind log with feet apart. Swing down to cut the side away from you (a). Do not chop downward (b).To split a small log, angle it against another log (c). Do not put your foot on it.

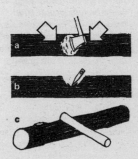

Broken handles: Axe handles break when the head misses the target and the handle takes the impact (a). To remove a broken handle, put it in a fire, burying metal in the earth to prevent it losing temper— single-headed (b), double-headed (c).

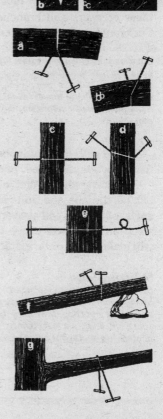

Using a flexible saw:
Always use a flexible saw so the cut opens (a) rather than closes (b), causing it to jam. Don't pull too hard or the saw will break. Keep the wire taut (c) pulling straight, never at angles (d). Maintain the rhythm when 2 people saw. A kink may break (e) the saw.

It is usually easier for a single person to cut a log by pulling it upward (f). Keep the log off the ground and give it an angle to keep cut open. Alternatively, to remove a branch, pull down from above (g). This could be dangerous. High branches can be removed by attaching strings to the saw toggles for extra reach. Be ready to jump clear of the branch.

FURNISHING THE CAMP

BEDS

Avoid lying on cold, damp ground. In the tropics raise the bed to provide a current of air. In cold climates, keep a fire going through the night and build a screen to reflect heat back on your sleeping area. On dry ground, stones heated in the fire and then buried under a thin layer of soil beneath the bedding will keep you warm.

A-Frame beds: Drive two pairs of posts into the ground at an angle, leaving a little more than your height between the pairs. Lash tops together. On hard ground cross-members will be needed between the feet of each A-frame and between the two A-frames.

Tube bed: Make a tube of strong material, sewn or thonged together. A large heavy-duty plastic bag is suitable. Do not use any fabric that might give under your weight or seams that might come apart.

Make A-frame supports, choose two straight poles, slightly longer than the distance between the frames, and pass them through the tube of fabric. Place them over the frames so they rest on the sides, the tube preventing them from slipping lower.

Bough bed: Fir-tree branches arranged in alternate layers make a comfortable and fragrant bed.

Ladder bed: Make A-frame supports and select poles as for the tube bed, and add a number of crosspieces. Strong, springy saplings are best. Lash end rungs to the

A-frame, jutting out either side. Make these of strong timber and lash them securely. Fit ladder over frames and lash in place. Lay bedding of ferns or leaves.

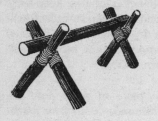

Seats: Never sit on damp ground. Use a log, or lash together a couple of low A-frame supports and rest a bough across them.

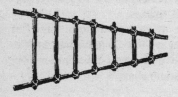

Ladder: Lash crosspieces to two long poles set at an angle, not parallel, so rungs won't slip down.

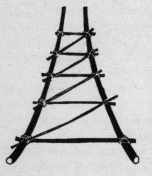

Travois: Choose two boughs with some spring to them and lash crosspieces, as for the ladder. Add additional struts to provide closer support. Pull the load on its runners like a sled. (See also p. 185.)

ANIMAL PRODUCTS

SKINS AND FURS

Properly prepared skins are supple, strong, and resist tearing. They have good thermal insulation, and are permeable to air and water vapor. For moccasins, shelters, laces, thongs, water bags or canoes, the fur is removed, but for warm clothing, bedding or a good insulating groundsheet it should be left on.

Remove fat and flesh by scraping the skin, using an edge of bone, flint or wood. Take care not to cut it. Remove every trace of flesh. Ants and other insects may help if you lay skin on the ground. Keep watch that they do not start to consume the skin itself.

To cure, stretch the skin as tight as possible and leave it in the sun to dry. Rubbing in salt or wood ash will aid the process. Do not let it get damp until the process is complete. If little or no sun is available, force-dry over a fire, but use only the heat and smoke and keep it away from the steam of any cooking pots.

Laces and lashings: Cut short laces straight from the skin, along its length. To obtain greater length cut in a spiral, keeping width consistent to avoid weak points.

Sinew as thread: The hamstring and the main sinews of the legs can be dried and used as thread, bowstrings, short ropes, and arrowhead bindings. They look like strong white cords. Sticky when wet, they dry hard.

Bladder: The bladder of a large animal can be used as a water carrier, as can the stomach. Tie off the openings to seal them.

CLOTHING

Salvage towels, blankets, seat-covers, curtains, sacking from the wreckage—any fabric can be used for garments, bedding or shelter.

Improve insulation by adding layers. Wear one sock on top of another and stuff dry grass or moss between them. Grass, paper, feathers, animal hair, etc., can be stuffed between other layers of clothing.

Use plastic bags and sheets to improvise waterproofs or cut off large sections of birch bark. Discard the outer bark and insert the inner layer under outer clothing.

Improve water-repellent qualities by rubbing animal fat or the tallow from suet into your clothing. Do not do this in situations of intense cold, where the reduction in insulation would be too great a loss.

Cut shoe soles from rubber tires, make holes around edges for thongs to tie them over wrapped feet, or to sew on to fabric uppers.

Tie on several layers of foot-wrappings with thongs or use a triangular shape. Fold one point back over toes, make slits in front. Bring other points from behind heel, through slits and tie around ankle.

Tie long leaf strips and fibers around a belt or neck band to hang down as a grass skirt or cape.

Cut a head hole in a blanket or carpet and use as a poncho. Tie at waist or thong sides.

Sew together small skins. Fur on the inside will give greater insulation but on outer garments the suede side sheds snow better.

ROPES AND LINES

Match the type, thickness and length of rope you carry to the demands you expect to make on it. Nylon has advantages in very damp climates and when weight is critical but can melt and is slippery when wet.

Rope about 9–10 mm (c. ½ in) is recommended for lashings, throwing and mountaineering. It can be used for safety lines and for climbing, provided belay and abseiling techniques are used—it is not thick enough for a hand over hand and foot grip.

Climbing rope must be elastic, to absorb shock without putting strain on anyone who falls.

TAKING CARE OF ROPE

Rope should be protected from exposure to damp or strong sunlight and, if made from natural fibers, from attack by rodents and insects.

If it does get wet, do not force-dry it in front of a fire. Do not drag it or leave it on the ground. Dirt can penetrate and work away at the fibers.

Try to keep rope for the job for which it was intended— do not use clothesline for climbing, or climbing rope for lashing—though in a survival situation you may have to use the same length of rope for many purposes.

THROWING A ROPE

A coil of rope is easier to throw than a loose end. Have a large knot or weight on the throwing end. Make sure that you keep hold of the other end! Always overthrow a lifeline so that the recipient stands a chance of catching part of the rope, even if they miss the end.

To throw a rope: Coil half the rope on fingers and palm of right hand, raise index finger and coil remainder on other fingers only. Pass second coil back to left hand. As you throw, release right-hand coil a split second before the left.

For a long throw: Tie a suitable missile to the end of the rope. Coil rope carefully on the ground or loop it loosely over the other hand so it will pay out freely.

Don't risk losing your end. Tie it to an anchor such as a heavy stone. Use a killick hitch (see p. 161).

If throwing a weighted rope over a branch, keep out of its path as it swings back toward the throwing point. If throwing a lifeline, make sure you don't knock out the person you're trying to help.

ROPE MAKING

Vines, grasses, rushes, barks, palms and animal hairs can all be used to make rope or line.

The stems of nettles make first-class ropes and those of honeysuckle can be twisted together to make tight lashings. The stronger the fiber, the stronger the rope. Some stiff fibers can be made flexible by steaming or warming. While pliable vines and other long plant stems can be used for short-term purposes, they may become brittle as they dry out. A rope made from plant fibers twisted ("spun") or plaited together will be more durable.

The tendons from animals' legs also make good strings, but they tend to dry hard. (They are also very useful as binding on arrow and spear heads; see pp. 83–84).

KNOTS

It is important to select the right knot for the task in hand. You never know when you may need to tie a knot, so learn their uses and how to tie—and untie—each one.

In the instructions for individual knots that follow the end of the rope or cord being used to tie the knot is referred to as the "live end" to distinguish it from the other end of the rope, or "standing part."

Reef knot: Use to tie ropes of same thickness. Holds firm under strain, yet is easily untied. It is not reliable for ropes of different diameters, nor for nylon. Can be tied in other materials—use in first aid. It will lie flat against the patient.

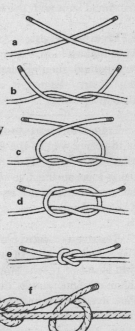

Pass right end over left (a) and then under it (b). Take left over right (c) and under it (d).

Check—the 2 loops should slide on each other. Tighten by pulling both strands on each side (e). To be doubly sure, finish by making a half-hitch with the live ends on either side of the knot (f).

SIMPLE KNOTS

These knots are quickly made and will help you understand the more complicated knots that follow.

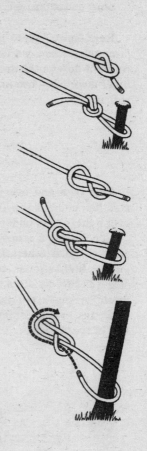

Overhand knot: Make a loop and pass the live end back through it.

Overhand loop: Fixed loop for throwing over a projection. Double the end of rope and tie overhand knot with the loop.

Figure-of-eight: An end-stop. Make a loop. Carry live end first behind, then around, standing apart. Bring it forward through the loop.

Figure-of-eight loop: Made in the same way as the figure-of-eight, but with line doubled, using loop as the live end. Can be used over a spike anchor for a belaying rope.

Rewoven figure-of-eight: Use when top end of a projection is out of reach. Make loose figure-of-eight along the rope. Pass live end around anchor and feed it back around the figure-of-eight, following exactly. Ease tight.

JOINING ROPES

Sheet bend: If correctly made and strain is not erratic this won't slip.

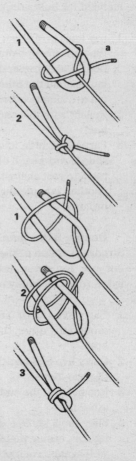

1 Make a loop in one rope. Take live end of the other (a) right around behind loop to the front, carry it over itself and then tuck down through loop.
2 Draw it tight and ease into shape as strain is increased.

Double sheet bend: More secure variation of sheet bend—use on wet ropes and where strain is not constant.

1 Make a loop in the thicker rope. Take live end of thinner rope (a) through loop, beneath thicker live end and then forward on outside of loop and right around it. Bring thin live end back between itself and outside of thick loop.
2 Take thin live end completely around the loop again and back through same place on outside of thick loop.
3 Draw tight and ease into shape.

If not tightened these knots tend to work loose. Do not use with smooth lines, e.g., nylon fishing line.

Fisherman's knot: Ideal for joining springy vines, wires, slippery lines and gut fishing line (soak gut first to make it pliable). Very secure but hard to untie. Not recommended for bulky ropes or nylon line.

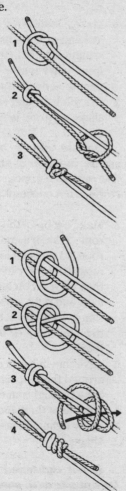

1 Lay lines beside each other, the ends in opposite directions. Carry live end of one line around the other and make a simple overhand knot.
2 Repeat with live end of other line.
3 Partially tighten knots and slide toward each other. Ease them to rest against one another, completing tightening process.

Double fisherman's:
Stronger version of the above. Do not use for nylon fishing lines, nylon ropes, or bulky ropes.

1 Carry live end of one line around the other, then around both.
2 Carry live end back through the two loops.
3 Repeat with the end of the other line.
4 Slide the 2 knots together and tighten, easing them to rest well against each other. Apply strain gradually.

Tape knot: Use to join flat materials, e.g., leather, webbing, tape and sheets or other fabrics.

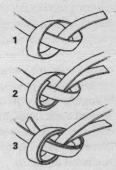

1 Make an overhand knot in the end of one tape. Do not pull it tight.
2 Feed the other tape through it so it follows exactly the shape of the first knot.
3 Live ends should be well clear of the knot so that they will not slip back when you tighten it.

Loop making

Bowline: A fixed loop that will neither tighten nor slip under strain. Use at the end of a lifeline.

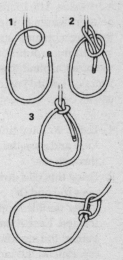

1 Make a small loop a little way along the rope.
2 Bring live end up through it, around standing part and back down through loop.
3 Pull on live end to tighten, easing knot into shape. Finish with a half-hitch.

Running bowline: A loop which tightens easily. Make a small bowline and pass long end of rope through loop.

Never tie a running bowline around the waist, it acts like a hangman's noose and could kill.

Triple bowline: A bowline made with a double line. Form a loop, pass doubled live end through loop, behind standing part and back through loop. This produces 3 loops which can be used for equipment haulage, or as a sit-sling or lifting harness with one loop around each thigh and the other around the chest. It takes practice—learn it before you need to use it.

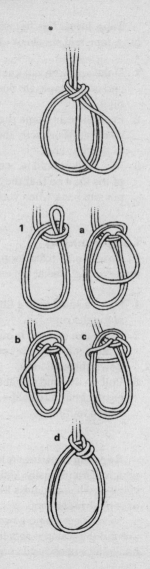

Bowline-on-the-bight: To support or lift someone from a crevasse. The loops will neither tighten nor jam, forming a bosun's chair, one loop fitting around buttocks, the other around upper body. Practice before you need to use it.

1 Using doubled line, form a loop and pass the live end through it.
2 Bring this end down (a) and over the end (b) of the larger double loop now formed. Ease it back up to behind the standing part (c). Pull on the large double loop to tighten (d).

Manharness hitch: A non-slip loop. It can be made along the length of the rope, but does not require access to an end. Several loops can be put on a rope for harnessing people together. Also a good way of preparing a rope for climbing. Toes and wrists can be put into the loops to carry weight, allowing you to take a rest.

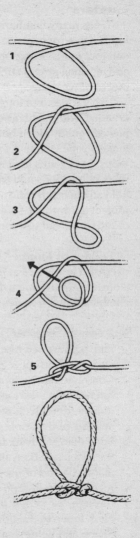

1 Make a loop in rope—look closely at the drawing.
2 Allow left side of rope to cross over loop.
3 Twist loop.
4 Pass it over left part of rope and through upper part of original loop.
5 Pull knot gently into shape, ease tight and test carefully.

Note: If not eased tight correctly loop may slip.

Different ways of making this knot may be found where the loop is not twisted at **3**. The final strength of the loop does not appear to be affected either by making this twist or not, nor if the twist should straighten out in use.

Ladders

Tie as many manharness hitches in a rope as you need hand and foot holds. Rungs may be added, using strong sticks or pieces of wreckage.

Use 2 ropes or a long rope, doubled, with manharness hitches placed equally along both sides to make a rope ladder. As you make loops, pass sticks through the corresponding loops and ease tight to hold sticks firmly. Allow sticks to project a few inches on either side of the ropes and test for strength.

Ladder of knots: A series of overhand knots tied at intervals along a smooth rope will make climbing it much easier.

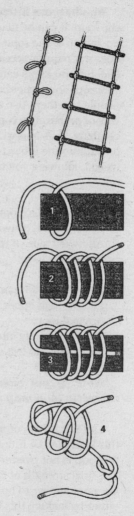

1 Leaving a reasonably long free end, make a half-hitch near the end of a short piece of log.
2 Continue making loose half-hitches along the log—the diameter of which will fix the spacing of the knots.
3 Pass start end back through all the loops and then slide them all off the end of the log.
4 As each turn of rope comes through, the center of the half-hitch loops to the other end. Shape and tighten each knot.

Honda knot: A free-running noose with a circular loop which is ideal for lassoing. If you have only one rope, don't use it as a lasso—this causes wear and damage to rope.

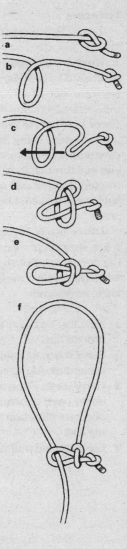

a Start with an overhand knot.
b Form a loop farther down the rope.
c Double rope into a bight between loop and knot.
d Pass bight through loop.
e Tighten loop around bight.
f Pass long end of rope through new eye formed by bight.

Before lassoing an animal, consider its strength. A big animal may wrench the rope away, depriving you of a meal and a rope. If the rope is anchored to you, you may be dragged along and injured. Instead, use a firm anchor—a tree or rock—to take the strain.

Hitches

Use to attach ropes to posts, bars and poles.

Round turn and two half-hitches: The best way to secure a rope to a post. Can take strain from any direction. Carry rope behind post, then around again. Bring live end over and back under standing end and through loop thus formed. Tighten and repeat half-hitch to make knot secure.

Clove hitch: Effective when strain is perpendicular to the horizontal. Not so good when the strain comes at an angle or is erratic.

1 Pass live end over and around bar.
2 Bring it across itself and around the bar again.
3 Carry the live end up and under itself, moving in the opposite direction to standing end.
4 Close up and pull tight.

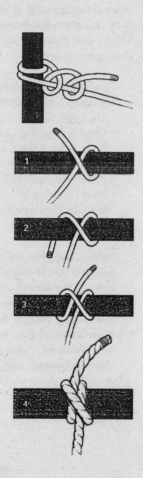

Timber hitch: Use as a start knot for lashings and for hoisting and for dragging or towing heavy logs.

1   Bring live end around bar and loosely around standing end.
2   Carry forward and tuck beneath rope encircling bar. Twist around as many times as comfortably fit. Tighten knot by gently pulling on standing end until a firm grip is achieved.

Killick hitch: To secure a line to an anchoring weight, make a timber hitch around one end of weight and tighten. Carry line along weight and make a half-hitch.

Marlin spike hitch: A temporary knot for securing a mooring line to a post, or for dragging over the top of an upright peg. By attaching a short, stout stick to the line it is possible to gain extra purchase for a firmer pull.

1   Form a loop in the rope—study drawing carefully.
2   Bring one side of loop back up over standing end.
3   Drop this over the pole—the pole coming between extended loop and standing part. Pull live end to tighten.

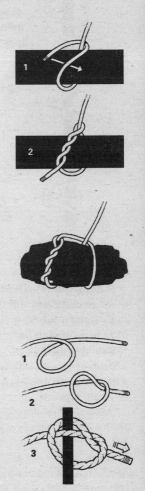

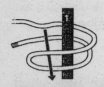

Quick-release knot: A secure knot, but will come untied with a single sharp tug on the live end. Recommended for temporarily anchoring lines.

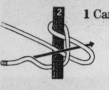

1 Carry a bight around a post or rail.

2 Bring a bight from the standing end through the first bight.

3 Form live end into a further bight and push doubled end through loop of second bight. Pull on standing end to tighten knot.

4 To release pull sharply on live end.

Shortening rope

Sheepshank: Treble the line. Form half-hitches in outer lengths and slip over adjoining bends. Or, instead of half-hitches, when a loop is formed in the standing part, pull a bight through it and

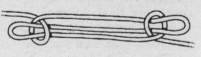

slip this over bend in rope. Tighten as you gradually increase tension.

Make a sheep-shank more secure by passing a stick through the bend

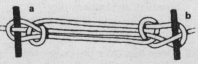

and behind the standing part (a). Or, if you have access to the rope's end, pass that through the bight (b). A stick would make this more secure.

> **Never cut a rope unnecessarily: a joined rope has only
> half the strength of a continuous one. Use sheepshank
> to shorten it or to exclude a damaged section.**

Securing loads

Wakos transport knot: Use to secure a high load or to
tie down a roof. For maximum purchase, pull down with
all your weight, then secure with 2 half-hitches. If it comes
loose, undo the hitches, retighten and secure.

1 Make a loop in rope.
   Farther down,
   toward end of rope,
   make a bight.
2 Pass bight through
   loop.
3 Make a twist in the
   new lower loop. Pass
   end of rope around
   securing point and
   up through this twist.
4 Pull end to tighten.
5 With end make two
   half-hitches around
   lower ropes to
   secure. Undo these
   to adjust and
   retighten.

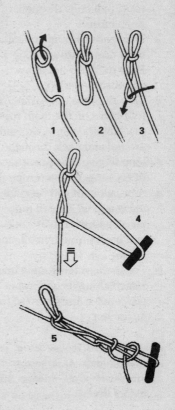

Prusik knot: A sliding loop. It will not slip under tension, but will slide along when tension is released. A pair of prusiks provide hand- and footholds for climbing or for swinging along a horizontal line. Slide them along main rope as you proceed. Also good for tent guylines.

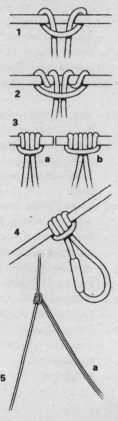

1 Pass a bight around main rope, pull ends through. Keep loose.
2 Take ends over again and back down through loop. Ease tight. Do not allow circuits to overlap.
3 This gives the appearance of four turns on the main rope (a). Mountaineers take ends around and back through loop to give the appearance of six turns on main rope (b).
4 A prusik knot can be made using a fixed spliced loop: pass bight over main rope and back through itself, and repeat.
5 For use as a tensioning line attach along the guy rope etc., and secure ends (a) to an anchor.

When used for climbing, or traveling along a rope, a spliced loop (4) is safest. If you have no spliced loop, join ends after knot is made. Test joins rigorously before use.

Lashings

Methods of lashing differ according to the position of the components. These techniques are invaluable in making rafts, shelters, etc.

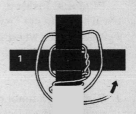

Square lashing: For lashing spars which cross at right angles.

1 Make a timber hitch carrying line alternately above and below both spars in a complete circuit before securing it. Then carry rope anticlockwise over and under both spars.

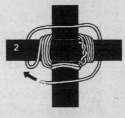

2 After three or four circuits make a full turn around a spar and circuit in the opposite direction.

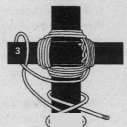

3 Complete circuits with a half-hitch around one spar and secure with a clove hitch on a spar at right angles.

Round lashing: Use to lash spars alongside each other or to extend length of a spar.

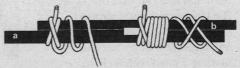

Begin with a clove hitch around both spars (a), then bind rope around them. Finish knot with a clove hitch at other end (b). Force a wedge under lashings to make them really tight. If spars are vertical bang the wedge in downward.

Diagonal lashing: Use when spars do not cross at right angles, or when spars need to be pulled toward one another for tying.

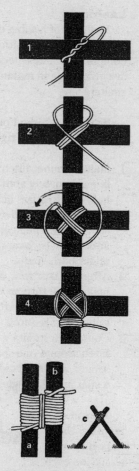

1 Begin with a timber hitch around both spars, placed diagonally.
2 Frap (lash) both spars with a few turns of rope over a timber hitch, then make a full turn under the bottom spar.
3 Frap across other diagonal, then bring rope back over one spar and make two or three circuits above upper spar and below lower.
4 Finish with a clove hitch on a convenient spar.

Shear lashing: To tie ends of two spars at an angle, e.g., for an A-frame. Begin with a clove hitch (a) around one spar. Bind, not very tightly, around both. Bring rope between spars and frap a few times around binding. Finish with a clove hitch around other spar (b). Tighten by opening up shears (c). A similar method can be used around three poles to make a tripod. Make turns around all three legs and frappings in the two gaps. The feet of A-frames and tripods should be anchored to stop them from spreading.

Fishing knots

Hook on to gut: Turl knot.
Soak gut. Thread through eye
of hook. Make overhand loop
and pass a bight through it (a)
to form a simple slip knot (b).
Pass hook through slip knot (c)
and pull tight around shank.

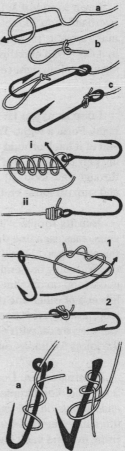

Hook on to nylon I: Half
blood knot. Thread end
through eye. Make 4 turns
around standing part. Pass live
end through loop formed next
to hook (i). Pull taut and snip
off fairly close to end (ii).

Hook on to nylon II: Two
turn turl knot. Thread hook.
Pass live end around standing
part to form a loop and through
it. Twist live end twice around
side of loop. Hold loop and pull
twists tight. Pass hook through
loop (1). Pull on standing part
to tighten loop on hook (2).

Jam knots: To secure
improvised hooks to gut or
cord. With an eye: thread gut.
Make two turns around hook and bring live end up
through turns (a). Ease tight and test for strength. Without
an eye: make loop around lower part of shaft. Make two
half-hitches from upper end downward and pass live end
through lower loop (b). Pull on standing part to tighten.

Loop in nylon I: Double overhand loop. Double line to make a bight. Tie an overhand in it (a). Twist end through again (b). Pull tight (c) and snip off end.

Loop in nylon II: Blood bight. Form a bight. Twist the end of it back around the standing part (i). Bring end back through new loop (ii). Pull tight and snip off loose end.

Joining loops: With free ends: pass each line through the other loop (1) and pull tight (2). With only one end free: make loop on one line. Take live end of other line through loop, around it and back through and then tie off with either of the knots for hooks on to nylon.

Joining nylon: Double three-fold blood knots. Place ends alongside and twist one three times around the other. Bring live end back and pass it through the space where the two lines cross over the other line and under its own standing end (a). Repeat in the opposite direction with the other line. Live ends then point in opposite directions (b). Ease tight.

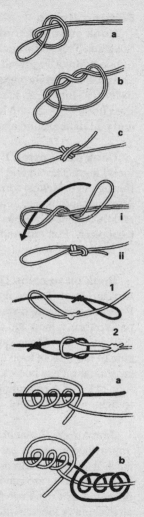

READING THE SIGNS

I N addition to being able to read and make a map, your survival depends on interpreting natural signs to help you find your way and to anticipate the weather.

MAPS

Choose your maps carefully. Make sure the scale is appropriate to your needs. Above all, make sure that you can interpret the information given.

INTERPRETING MAPS

Altitude: Since height cannot be reproduced on paper, altitudes are recorded as contour lines, representing a series of points at the same distance above sea level. However, they do not record what happens in between.

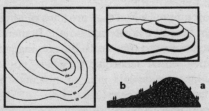

Closely grouped contours indicate a steep slope (a). Greater spaces between contour lines show gentler inclines (b). The rise in the ground is not comparable to the scale of the distance shown between them (on a 1:50,000 map, contours at 5 mm would indicate a gradient of 1 in 25).

Scale: The scale of a typical walker's map is 1:50,000, i.e., each measure represents a distance 50,000 times greater on the ground. Not all features can be shown to scale: roads, paths, streams and rivers are usually given standardized widths. Study the key and master the way information is presented—which symbols represent which features (swamps, woodlands, buildings).

Coordinates: Map grids are based either on degrees of latitude and longitude or on ground measurements. For example, on British Ordnance Survey maps, grid lines represent areas 1 km apart with the diagonal across them 1.5 km. A position can be described by a coordinate made up from the line references from two adjoining sides of the map. This provides an easy way of telling rescuers of your location or fixing a rendezvous point.

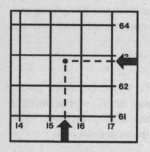

The point marked with a dot can be described as 15.5 x 62.8 using the coordinates from the sides of this grid. The map reference is usually expressed as 6 digits: 155628. Any letter area codes on the map should be included.

North on maps: Unless they are lines of longitude, grid lines do not indicate north and south. Remember that a compass points not to true north but to magnetic north—the difference varies according to where you are in the world. If your map doesn't indicate magnetic north, you can find it from the Pole Star (see p. 176).

In the northern hemisphere point the compass at the Pole Star. Note the difference between the pointer and indicated north. Line the compass up with the grid lines on the map to discover their variation. If you propose to walk on magnetic bearings you must compensate for the variation. If unable to make appropriate corrections, continually check your position against visible features.

Measuring distances: As-the-crow-flies distances can be measured using a straight edge, which is then matched against the scale. Gradients make a difference. For example, a gradient of 45° will add another 82 m to a horizontal map distance of 200 m (500 ft to 725 ft).

Your own maps: If you do not have a map, make one. Find the best vantage point and study the terrain. Note the number and direction of ridges—you won't be able to see what lies between them, so leave gaps to be filled in as you gain information from other vantage points.

Mark anything of interest on your map: watercourses, rocky outcrops, landmarks, areas of vegetation. Plot positions of your traps, animal lairs, and places for foraging for food, fuel and stones for implements. It will be much easier than relying on your memory.

DIRECTION FINDING

The sun rises in the east and sets in the west, roughly speaking. In the northern hemisphere, at noon, the sun will be due south; in the southern hemisphere it will be due

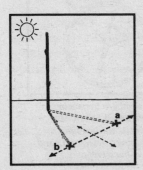

north. The hemisphere is indicated by the way shadows move: clockwise in the north, anticlockwise in the south.

Shadow stick method 1: Place a 1 m (3 ft) stick upright on a patch of flat ground. Mark where tip of shadow falls (a). Wait 15 minutes and mark new shadow tip (b). Join the two for the directions of east and west—first mark is west. North–south are at right angles to line.

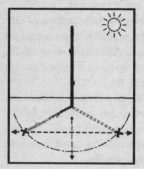

Shadow stick method 2: Mark first shadow tip in morning. Draw an arc at exactly this distance from the tip, using stick as center point. Shadow shrinks at midday. In the afternoon, as shadow lengthens, mark the exact spot where it touches arc. Join to give east and west—west is the morning mark.

Direction by watch: A traditional analogue watch with two hands can tell direction, provided it is set to true local time (ignoring daylight saving and conventional time zones). The nearer the Equator you are, the less accurate this method is.

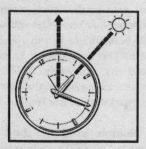

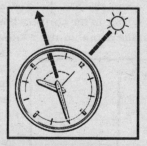

In northern hemisphere, hold watch horizontal. Point hour hand at sun. Bisect angle between hour hand and 12 mark to give north–south line.

In southern hemisphere, hold watch horizontal. Point 12 toward sun. Mid-point between 12 and hour hand will give a north–south line.

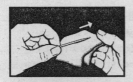

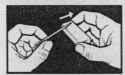

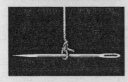

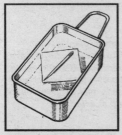

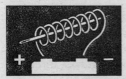

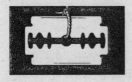

Improvised compasses: A piece of ferrous metal wire (a sewing needle is ideal) stroked repeatedly in one direction against silk will become magnetized and can be suspended so it points north.

Stroking with a magnet will be better than using silk—stroke the metal smoothly from one end to the other in one direction only.

Suspend the needle in a loop of thread so balance is not affected. Kinks or twists in thread must be avoided.

A floating needle can be used in the same way as the suspended one above. Lay the needle on a piece of paper, bark or grass and float it on the surface of water.

A power source of 2 volts or more, e.g., a battery, can be used with a short length of insulated wire to magnetize metal. Coil wire around needle. If the wire is uninsulated, wrap needle with paper or cardboard. Attach ends of wire to battery terminals for 5 minutes.

A razor blade can also be used as a compass needle. Magnetize the blade by stropping with care against palm of hand, then suspend.

Use other methods to establish the general direction of north, then mark the relevant end of your new "compass" to indicate north. Top up your needle's magnetism from time to time, and always check readings against the sun.

PLANT POINTERS

Plants can give an indication of north and south. They tend to grow toward the sun, so flowers and most abundant growth will be to the south in the northern hemisphere, to the north in the southern. Moss on tree trunks will be greener and more profuse on that side.

If trees have been felled, the pattern of the rings is more widely spaced on the side toward the Equator.

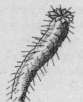

A South African plant, the north pole plant, leans toward the north.

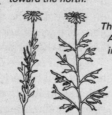

The compass plant is North American and directs its leaves in a north–south alignment so that profile from east or west is quite different from that of north or south.

Wind direction: If the direction of the prevailing wind is known it can be used to maintain direction.

Where a strong wind always comes from the same direction, plants and trees may be bent that way. Birds and insects will usually build nests on the leeside.

DIRECTION BY THE HEAVENS

Using the moon

As the moon orbits the earth over 28 days, the shape varies according to its position. When it is on the same side of the earth as the sun, no light is reflected from the sun (a): this is the new moon. Then it reflects light on its apparent right-hand side in a gradually increasing area as it waxes. At the full moon it is on the opposite side of the earth from the sun (b) and then it wanes, the reflecting area reducing to a narrow sliver on the apparent left-hand side.

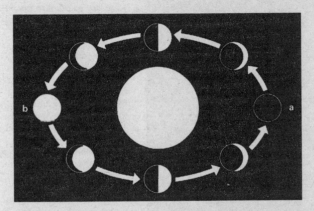

If the moon rises before the sun has set, the illuminated side will be on the west. If it rises after midnight the illuminated side will be the east. Thus the moon gives a rough east–west reference in the night.

Using the stars

The stars stay in the same relation to one another. Their passage over the horizon starts 4 minutes earlier each night—a 2-hour difference over a month.

In the northern hemisphere groups of stars remain visible throughout the night, wheeling around the only star that does not seem to move: the Pole Star (a useful navigation aid, located almost above polar north).

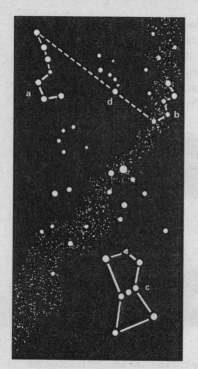

The northern sky:

The Plough or Big Dipper (a), Cassiopeia (b) and Orion (c) all circle the Pole Star (d), but (a) and (b) are recognizable groups that do not set. Use them to find the Pole Star.

Of the seven stars which form the Plough (a), the two lowest ones point to the Pole Star, about four times farther away than the distance between them.

Cassiopeia (b) is W-shaped, on the opposite side of the Pole Star and the same distance away as the Plough. On clear, dark nights this overlays the Milky Way. The center star points toward the Plough. A line can be drawn connecting Cassiopeia and the Plough through the Pole Star.

Orion (c) rises above the Equator and can be seen in both hemispheres. It rises on its side, due east and sets due west. It is farther from the Pole Star than Cassiopeia and the Plough.

Other stars that rise and set can be used to indicate direction. Set 2 stakes in the ground, one shorter than the other. Sight along them at any star except the Pole Star. From the star's apparent movement you can deduce direction in which you are facing:

Apparently rising = facing east
Apparently falling = facing west
Looping flatly to right = facing south
Looping flatly to left = facing north

These are only approximate directions. They will be reversed in the southern hemisphere.

The southern sky: There is no equivalent of the Pole Star near the South Celestial Pole, but the Southern Cross, a constellation of five stars, provides a signpost to south. It can be distinguished from two other cross-shaped groups by its smaller size and its two pointer stars. Look along the Milky Way for a dark patch (the Coal Sack); the Southern Cross is on one side of it.

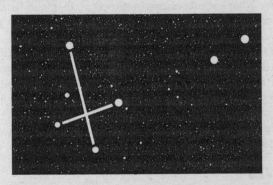

To locate south, project an imaginary line along the cross and four and a half times longer, then drop it vertically down to the horizon. Fix, if you can, a prominent landmark on the horizon, or drive two sticks into the ground, to help you find the position by day.

WEATHER SIGNS
Weather is much more localized than climate and there can be marked variations between one small area and the next.

COASTAL AREAS
A regular pattern of day–night change in wind direction suggests a large body of water—whether an ocean, inland sea or a lake—in the direction from which the day wind

blows (during the day breezes blow from the sea to the land; at night the wind changes and blows off the land).

WINDS

Certain scents—the smell of the sea or of vegetation—carried on the wind can provide information about the place from which they blow.

Study wind and weather patterns: wind from a certain direction is likely to bring similar weather each time it blows. Where winds maintain direction, they can be an aid in keeping to a course—but verify your course by other means at regular intervals.

If a wind is strong and dry the weather should remain constant until the wind drops or veers, then it may rain.

If it is foggy and misty you may get condensation but you will not get rain. However, if a wind rises and blows away the fog, it may turn to rain.

On a fine day a noticeable increase in the strength of the wind indicates an imminent weather change (see pp. 279–284).

CLOUDS

Clouds are the most reliable of weather signs. There are ten main types of cloud formation. Approximate altitudes are given for each type. The same shapes occur at lower altitudes in polar regions. The higher the clouds, the finer the weather. The figures given at the end of the following entries indicate cloud heights.

 Cirrocumulus clouds: Look like rippled sand. An omen of fair weather, they usually follow a storm and dissipate to leave a clear blue sky.

 Altocumulus clouds: Fair-weather clouds, on a larger scale than cirrocumulus, thicker, not so white and with shadows in them. Usually appear after a storm.

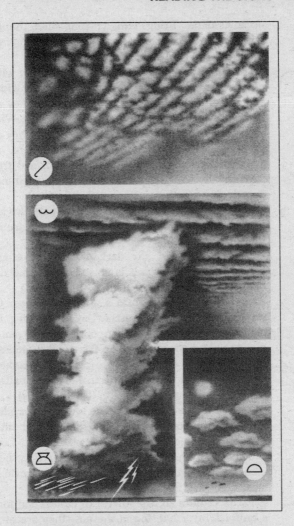

Cumulonimbus clouds: Low thunder clouds.
Dark and menacing, with the top flattening out in

an anvil shape. Brings hail, a strong wind, thunder and lightning. False cirrus appear above them, false nimbostratus below.

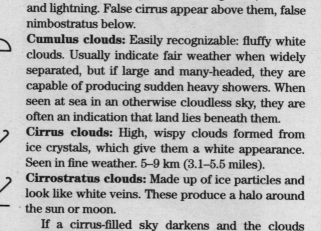

Cumulus clouds: Easily recognizable: fluffy white clouds. Usually indicate fair weather when widely separated, but if large and many-headed, they are capable of producing sudden heavy showers. When seen at sea in an otherwise cloudless sky, they are often an indication that land lies beneath them.

Cirrus clouds: High, wispy clouds formed from ice crystals, which give them a white appearance. Seen in fine weather. 5–9 km (3.1–5.5 miles).

Cirrostratus clouds: Made up of ice particles and look like white veins. These produce a halo around the sun or moon.

If a cirrus-filled sky darkens and the clouds change to cirrostratus it is an indication that rain or snow is on the way. 5–9 km (3.1–5.5 miles).

Altostratus clouds: Form a grayish veil over the sun or moon. If wet weather is approaching the cloud will darken and thicken, obscuring the sun or moon until it begins to rain. 2.5–6 km (1.6–3.7 miles).

Nimbostratus clouds: Form low, dark blankets, which signal rain or snow within 4–5 hours, usually lasting several hours. 1.5–5 km (0.9–3.1 miles).

Stratocumulus clouds: Form a low, lumpy, rolling mass, usually covering the whole sky, though often thin enough for the sun to filter through. Light showers may precipitate from them, but these clouds usually dissipate in the afternoon, leaving a clear night sky. Below 2.5 km (1.6 miles).

Stratus clouds are the lowest of clouds and form a uniform layer like fog in the air—they are often described as hill fog. Although not a normal rain cloud, they can produce drizzle. When they form

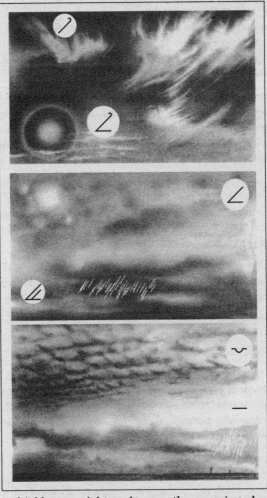

thickly overnight and cover the morning sky they will usually be followed by a fine day. Less than 2.5 km (1.6 miles).

WEATHER PREDICTION

To be caught in bad weather could prove fatal. Before setting out, take note of the weather. Observe wind and pressure changes. Keep a record of the weather, the conditions which precede it, and what they develop into.

Animals are sensitive to atmospheric pressure and are good for short-term weather predictions. Insect-eating birds feed higher in good weather, lower when a storm is approaching. Unusual rodent activity during the day may be a prelude to bad weather.

Humans can sometimes sense a change in the weather, too. Curly-haired people find their hair becomes tight and unmanageable as bad weather approaches. Those with rheumatism, corns or similar ailments suffer discomfort in wet weather.

If camp fire smoke rises steadily, the weather is likely to remain fine. If it starts swirling, or is beaten down after rising a short way, a storm or shower is coming.

Sounds carry farther when wet weather is on the way and the smell of vegetation becomes more distinctive before the arrival of rain.

A red sky at night means that there is little moisture in the atmosphere and rain is unlikely within the next two hours. A red sky in the morning indicates a storm is approaching. A gray morning heralds a dry day, and a gray evening sky means that rain is imminent.

A *corona*, a colored circle visible around the sun or moon, will enlarge if fair weather lies ahead and shrink if rain is likely. A rainbow in the late afternoon is another sign of good weather.

ON THE MOVE

THIS section deals with skills needed on the move. It should be read in conjunction with the techniques described in *Climate and Terrain* (p. 24).

THE DECISION TO MOVE

In the short term, unless local dangers or a lack of food and water make it imperative to leave the site of your accident, stay close in the hope of rescue. If you have injured persons and limited resources, send a party to contact help while others stay to care for the sick.

In the long term, if no rescue comes, resources may become exhausted and there is an increased risk of disease from staying too long in one place. Such factors will make a move advisable.

Where to go next will be determined by the information you have been able to gather, by the fitness and endurance of the group and the nature of the terrain. Remember: the most direct route may not be the easiest to travel.

If you have a clear idea of your location, make for the nearest settlement. If you have no idea where you are, follow waterways downstream—they generally lead to populated areas. Move at least three days' journey from the old camp so that fuel, flora and fauna will be undisturbed in the new location.

Before you abandon camp, leave signs to show you have moved on (see p. 220), and where you are heading. Rescuers can then follow you.

PREPARATIONS

Stock up preserved food, and make water containers.

Make foot-coverings and clothing, and packs to carry equipment and supplies. Build a sledge or raft or other form of transport.

Take signaling gear and shelter materials with you. If shelter can be quickly erected on arrival you will then be free to gather food and fuel.

Study weather patterns. Set off in settled weather.

Hudson bay pack: A comfortable and simple way to carry equipment, this needs strong, waterproof material c.

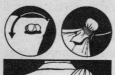

90 cm (1 yd) square, two small stones and cord or thong long enough to loop across the body.

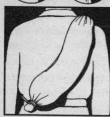

Place stones in diagonally opposite corners of the cloth. Fold ends of cloth over stones. Tie cord below stones to secure them in position—they will prevent cord slipping off. Lay cloth on ground and roll possessions up tightly. Wrap pack around body, either across the back or around the waist.

Carry babies papoose-style on your back or front. Tie lower corners of a rectangle of cloth around the waist, pop in baby and tie upper corners around your neck.

Sit small children on a backpack frame. For adults and heavy equipment make a travois (see p. 146) or sledge.

MAKING A SLEDGE

Ideal for snow and ice, sledges may also be used on smooth ground. Use doors and cowlings from a crashed vehicle or plane in construction. Tie lines to front runners with a bowline to the people hauling—ideally two at the front and two at the rear. Test before use.

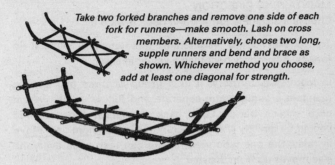

Take two forked branches and remove one side of each fork for runners—make smooth. Lash on cross members. Alternatively, choose two long, supple runners and bend and brace as shown. Whichever method you choose, add at least one diagonal for strength.

PLANNING THE ROUTE

Visibility will often be restricted and you must guess what lies ahead. Things you can see may be misleading: what looks like an easy slope may prove to be a barrier when you get close. If you have them, use binoculars.

Climbing a tree may help you see farther, but keep close to the trunk and test each branch before risking your weight on it. This is no time to risk a fall.

FOLLOWING RIVERS

Watercourses offer a route to civilization and a life-support system on the way. Apart from rare occasions when they suddenly disappear underground, rivers offer a clearly defined route. Where they cut through gorges it may be impossible to follow their banks—take to high ground and cut off the bends.

In tropical conditions, vegetation may be densest by the

river and the banks hard to negotiate. If the river is wide enough, build a raft of bamboo or fallen trees.

When a river meanders widely on a plain the inside of loops may be swampy and prone to flooding. Avoid these marshy areas if you can—cut across the loop.

MAINTAINING DIRECTION

Choose a distant landmark and head toward it.

Try to skirt dense vegetation: orientation is difficult in forests. A compass becomes a valuable asset.

In featureless territory, if in a group of three or more, to maintain a straight line separate and follow at intervals in each other's tracks. Look back frequently: those behind should be directly behind each other in a straight line. Move in relay: the one who went ahead can rest while everyone else moves up from the rear.

If traveling alone, align yourself by looking back at your own tracks, if visible, or set up markers (sticks, piles of stones) at intervals in alignment with each other so you can check that you are not deviating from your route.

Once on high ground, stick to it until certain that you have found the spur down which will allow you to make the best progress in the desired direction.

MOVING IN GROUPS

Always move in formation. This will make it easy to check that no stragglers have been left behind. Have a briefing before setting out to discuss the route and to designate rallying points at which to regroup.

DIVIDING RESPONSIBILITIES

Appoint a scout to select the best route and find ways to skirt obstacles. A number two should make sure the scout maintains correct overall direction. Both will need to be relieved frequently as it is tiring work.

The others should travel in pairs to ensure that no one drops by the wayside. A head count is vital after negotiating difficult terrain (check equipment regularly too). Nominate prominent landmarks as rallying points so that everyone knows what to head for if separated.

PACE AND PROGRESS

A large group can send an advance party to clear the route and set up camp. A clear trail will make carrying baggage and injured people much easier.

The scout must not go too fast. Frequent rests—a 10-minute break every 30–45 minutes—are vital. After an obstacle wait and allow everyone to catch up and check and adjust loads.

Try to maintain an even pace. A smooth, pendulum-like movement is easiest. Keep arms free to aid balance. On steep ground the pace should be shortened, on easy ground lengthened. Avoid overstepping on descents. Use ropes to provide handholds on slippery terrain. Attach prusik knots (see p. 164) for extra safety.

WALKING AT NIGHT

Negotiating territory at night can be dangerous, but may be necessary. Because it is difficult to see clearly you are easily disoriented. It is always darker among trees, so keep to open country if you can. When looking at an object at night, look at one side rather than directly at it. It is hard to distinguish anything in a dark mass, but edges show clearly.

It takes 30–40 minutes for the eyes to get accustomed to darkness. Once this is achieved, protect eyes from bright light or night vision will be impaired. If a light

must be used, cover one eye so that vision in that eye
will be retained. A red filter over a torch will also help.

Ears are good sensors. The sound of a river indicates
how fast it flows. Smells can aid identification.

Walk slowly. Test each step before putting your weight
forward. Use a shuffling step to descend slopes.

UPLAND TRAVEL

In mountainous country keep to high ground—it makes
navigation easier. Rivers in steep-sided gullies are difficult
to negotiate on foot: climb up and follow the ridges. Drop
down to collect water and to seek shelter, but don't go
right to the valley bottom if you can find what you need on
the way. Pockets of cold air get trapped in valley bottoms:
you may be warmer and less tired if you choose a sheltered spot higher up. If you carry water and shelter materials, stay on the high ground and make camp in a sheltered
spot. When the river gets larger and the valley opens out,
drop down to follow the riverbanks once more.

STEEP SLOPES

Traverse slopes in a zigzag. As you change direction always
set off with the uphill foot to avoid crossing your legs over
and losing balance. When climbing steep slopes, lock your
knees together after each step to rest the muscles.

To descend slopes, keep your knees bent and try to go
straight down (sit back and dig in the heels if you pick up
too much speed). Avoid loose rock and scree. When climbing, test every foothold before putting your weight on it.
Avoid stepping on stones or logs that may dislodge.

Jump down loose ground provided there are no sudden
drops. Keep feet square and shoulder-width apart, dig in
heels and slide. You will lose control as speed increases—
jump again. Abseil down steep slopes (see p. 33).

JUNGLE TRAVEL

You may have to cut through dense jungle if there is no way around. Chop downward and as low as possible at the stems on both sides so they fall away from the path, not across it. Avoid leaving bamboo spikes—they can be lethal if stumbled on. Atap and rattan have thorns like fish hooks at the end of the leaf. When snared, back off and untangle. Rushing only makes it worse.

> Keep feet covered to protect them from sapling spikes, snakes and chigoes (chiggers), burrowing parasites. Stop frequently to remove parasites. Chigoes ignored for more than an hour will cause infection.

WATERWAYS

A wide river will be easier to float on than to walk beside. Long-term survivors should experiment with making canoes by burning out the center of a tree trunk or covering a frame of willow with birch bark or skins.

RAFTS

A raft, even if the structure is not perfect, will not readily capsize.

Use bamboo, uprooted trees which are sound and unrotted, or the tops of the trunks of deadfalls. Oil drums or floating objects will support a raft. If there is no supply of timber a sheet of waterproof material can be used as a man-carrying coracle.

> Never take chances. Only a really tough structure will survive rapids, and on wide reaches you face a long swim to the bank if your raft breaks up. Test all rafts in safe water near camp before setting off on a journey.

Tie all equipment securely to the raft or safety line.

Make sure that nothing trails over the edges—it could snag in shallows.

Everyone aboard should have a bowline around the waist securing them to a safety line or to the raft. Lifelines should be long enough to allow free movement, but not so long as to trail in the water. In swift-flowing rivers with rapids and falls it is better not to tie on. Head for the bank if the raft is out of control.

In shallow water, control the raft with two long poles like a punt—one person poling at the front corner, another at the diagonally opposite back corner.

Bamboo raft: Cut thick-ish bamboo in 3 m (10 ft) lengths. Make holes through canes near ends and halfway along. Pass stakes through holes to connect canes. Lash each cane to the stakes with twine or vines. Make a second layer to fit on top of the first and lash them together.

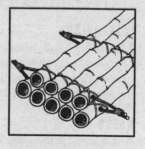

Gripper bar raft: Place two thickish, pliable stakes on the ground—they should be long enough to overlap the width of the deck. Lay logs over them. Place two stakes on top. Tie each pair of stakes on one side. Then, with a helper standing on top to force the other ends together, tie these so the logs are gripped between. Notch-

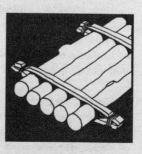

ing the ends of the gripper bars will stop ropes slipping.

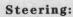

Steering:
Make a paddle
rudder and mount it on an A-frame
near one end of raft. Secure A-frame
with guylines to the corners of the
raft. Tie the rudder on so it does not
slip. You may need to notch the raft
for the A-frame base.

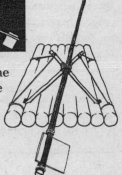

TRAVELING BY RAFT

A large group will need several rafts. The first should carry
no equipment or provisions, just the fittest group members
to act as lookouts and warn of hazards.

Waterfalls and rapids are often indicated by spray or mist.
They can also be heard for some distance. If in doubt, moor
the raft and reconnoiter on foot.

Unload the raft when you reach a dangerous stretch. Carry
equipment overland downstream and post someone at the
point where the river becomes safe to recover the raft. Then
go back and release the raft to drift down. It may need
repairs, but you will be safe.

Never raft in the dark. At night secure the raft firmly and
make shelter on high ground away from the river.

BOGS, MARSHES AND QUICKSAND

Avoid crossing a marsh if possible. If unavoidable, jump
from tuft to tuft. Should you sink in a bog, swim with a
breaststroke to firm ground. Don't try to jump. Spreading your body distributes your weight.

CROSSING RIVERS

River headwaters are narrow and swift-flowing. Find a place where water is shallow enough to wade across—test for hidden depths with a pole. Look for stepping stones, but mind you don't slip and sprain an ankle.

Estuaries have strong currents and are subject to tides. Avoid crossing there unless equipped with a boat or raft. Head upstream to find a safer spot. Do not set off right opposite the point you hope to reach—make allowances for where the current will take you.

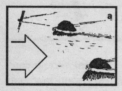

Study the water:
Surface movement can indicate what lies beneath. The main flow of the current is evident from a chevron shape of smoother water around any projection (a), the V widening downstream.

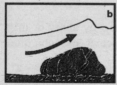

Waves that seem to stay in one position (b) are evidence of a boulder on the bottom.

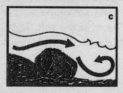

An obstruction close to the surface creates an eddy downstream where surface water appears to run back against the main flow. If a large boulder coincides with a steep drop (c) these eddies can produce a powerful backward pull downstream of the obstruction. They are very dangerous.

☠ ICE-COLD WATER IS A KILLER
Do not swim or wade through deep water at very low temperatures, it could prove fatal. Make a raft. Wade only if no more than your feet will get wet, and dry them vigorously as soon as you reach the other bank.

Wading across

Never underestimate a stretch of water, however shallow. Use a stick to aid balance. Roll trousers up or take them off so you have them dry for the other side. Keep boots on—they give a better grip than bare feet. Undo the belt fastening of a backpack so you can slip it off if you get swept over, but don't let go of it: use it to help you right yourself.

Turn at a slight angle, sideways on to your destination. The current will then take you there. Do not stride: shuffle sideways, using the stick to test for depth and trying each foothold before using it.

A group wading across together should line up behind the strongest, each holding the one in front at the waist and moving in step. Alternatively, link arms side-by-side, holding on to a branch or pole to keep in alignment. Cross facing the bank and moving forward. Only the side of the first person opposes the current and the group provides stability for everyone.

> ☠ Look out for submerged branches. You could get tangled and lose your balance. When forced against an obstruction by the current you feel its full force and may be unable to move.

Crossing with ropes

You need a loop of rope three times as long as the width of the stream and at least three people in the party—the fittest person crosses while two control the rope to keep it out of the water as much as possible, and stand by to haul the crosser to safety if difficulties are encountered.

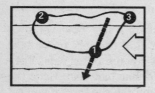

The person crossing is secured around the chest to the loop. The other two are not tied on. They pay out rope as it is needed. The strongest should cross first.

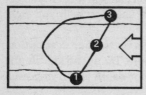

When he reaches the bank, 1 unties himself and 2 ties on and crosses, controlled by the others. Any number can be sent across this way.

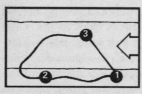

When 2 has reached the bank, 3 ties on and crosses. 1 takes most of the strain; 2 stands by in case anything goes wrong.

RIVERS ARE DANGEROUS

Never enter the water unless there is no other way of getting across. Choose a crossing point carefully.

Avoid high banks that are difficult to climb out on to.

Avoid obstructions in the water.

Current is likely to be fastest on the outside of bends, and steep banks may be undercut, making landing impossible.

Look for an even section of riverbed—shingle is the best surface for wading.

Swimming across

If you can't swim, don't try—rely on others and use a float. Even strong swimmers should use flotation aids to save energy and keep kit dry. Don't swim fully clothed, you need something warm to put on at the other end.

Make sure your landing point has a beach or something to haul yourself out with. Avoid tangled branches in the water where you might get trapped. Enter well upstream and let the current carry you.

Check the strength of the current by watching floating logs and flotsam. Look for obstructions and eddies. If you hit weed in the water, adopt a crawl stroke to cut through it. Once a strong swimmer has cleared a passage, others may follow in that channel.

FLOTATION AIDS

Use anything that floats: fuel cans, plastic bottles, logs.

Put your clothes in a waterproof bag, leaving plenty of air space. Tie the neck, bend it over and tie again. Hold on to it, using just your legs to propel yourself.

Pile twigs and straw into the center of a waterproof sheet to create air pockets, then pile your clothes and equipment on top and tie securely. Do not attempt to sit on the bundles or place your weight on them.

A group should split into fours, each lashing their bags together and using them as a support for an injured person or a nonswimmer.

If no waterproof material is available, make a small raft or coracle to float your things on. Bundle your belongings and, if heavy, make the raft two-layered so only the lower layer sinks and your kit stays dry.

SURVIVAL AT SEA

FOUR-FIFTHS of the earth's surface is open water—the most difficult environment in which to survive. Water and wind rapidly chill the body. Alone in cold water your chances are not good without equipment. If you know your location you may be able to predict where the currents will carry you. Warm currents, e.g., the Gulf Stream, are often rich in sea foods, as are coastal waters. Your main problem is likely to be a shortage of fresh water if you have no means of distilling seawater.

ABANDONING SHIP

When you are on board a ship, lifeboat drill should be a well-rehearsed procedure. Even in small boats everyone on board should be acquainted with safety equipment and procedures.

If the signal is given to abandon ship, put on warm, preferably woolen, clothing, including hat and gloves, and wrap a towel around your neck. Take a torch, chocolates and boiled sweets if you can. Don't panic. An orderly embarkation will be faster and will establish a calmer attitude. Take what equipment you can with you. A lifejacket will make it easier to float.

Don't inflate your lifejacket until you leave ship. On small boats lifejackets should be worn all the time. If you have to jump overboard, first throw something that floats and jump close to it. Without a lifejacket or belt, air trapped in clothing will aid buoyancy—a good reason to keep your clothes on despite the frequent advice to strip off before entering the water.

If you are swept overboard keep afloat and try to attract attention. Sound travels well over water—shout and splash. Wave with one arm above water (not both, you will go under). Movement makes you more noticeable. Most lifejackets are equipped with a whistle and light.

IN THE WATER

Swim slowly and steadily. If abandoning a sinking boat or aircraft get upwind and stay clear of it. Keep away from any fuel slick. If forced to swim through flames, jump in feet first and upwind. Swim into the wind using breast-stroke. Splash flames away from head to make breathing holes. Swim underwater until clear of danger. If an under-water explosion is likely, reduce the risk of injury by swimming on your back.

If within sight of land, relax and float until the ebb turns and helps carry you to land.

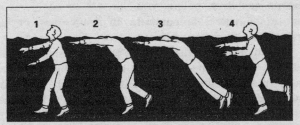

1 In rough seas, float upright and take a deep breath. **2** Lower face into water (keeping mouth closed) and bring arms forward to rest at water level. **3** Relax in this position until you need to take in more air. **4** Raise head above surface, tread water, and exhale. Take a breath and return to the relaxed position.

Flotation "bags": Improvise a short-term float from a pair of trousers. Knot bottoms of legs, sweep them over the head to fill with air, then hold the waist below water to trap the air, making legs into water wings.

Immediate action: Once clear of the wreck, inflate your dinghy. If there is no dinghy, grab as much flotsam as possible to use as a raft. Tie it together with belts, shoelaces, spare clothing. Salvage floating equipment.

Inflating a dinghy

Many dinghies are self-inflating. If not, a pump is provided. Dinghies are built in sections, so there are several inflation points.

Boarding an inflatable dinghy: If already in the water move to the end (not the side) of the dinghy, place one leg over the edge and roll into the vessel. Do not jump in from above, you may damage it. Large dinghies have a righting line attached to one side. Grab it from the opposite side, brace your feet against the dinghy and pull. The dinghy should rise up and over, pulling you out of the water momentarily. In heavy seas, or high winds, this can be very difficult.

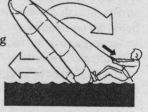

To haul someone else aboard, hold their shoulders and lift one leg over the end, then roll them in. Discourage them from putting their arms around your neck—they could pull you into the water. Then tie yourself and others to the dinghy.

Ensure the dinghy is fully inflated. It should be firm but not rock-hard. If not, inflate it with your own breath or a pump. The valves are one-way and air will not escape when you take off the protective cap.

Check for leaks. Escaping air causes bubbles under water and a hissing sound above water. Seal holes with screw-in conical plugs in the dinghy kit. There should also be a supply of rubber patches and adhesive.

Make daily checks for inflation and leaks. To repair a leak on the underside, swim under and insert a plug.

SURVIVAL AFLOAT

Rafts, boats and dinghies are built to carry a limited number. These numbers should not be exceeded.

Place infants and the infirm aboard, and as many able-bodied as can be accommodated. The rest must hang on in the water, frequently swapping places with fit survivors in the raft.

Stow gear in stowage places and tie securely. Check that no sharp objects will damage the inflatable. Put items that will spoil if wet in a waterproof container.

Check signaling equipment: heliographs, flares, etc.

If distress signals have been sent giving your position, try to maintain location. A sea anchor streamed out from the boat will keep it into the weather and slow down drift. Improvise a sea anchor from any weighted object securely tied to a line. Use clothing tied to a paddle with reef knots.

If you can see the shore head toward it.

SURVIVAL PRIORITIES

PROTECTION from weather and effects of exposure.
LOCATION Try to establish where you are and the best way of attracting rescue.
WATER Take stock. Ration at once. Collect rain.
FOOD Don't eat, unless you have sufficient water. Check all rations, stow them securely. Start fishing.

PROTECTION

Keep a log: record names of survivors; date, time, and position of accident; weather conditions; equipment salvaged. Record sightings and circumstances daily.

In a cold climate: Get out of cold water as soon as possible. Keep the dinghy as dry as you can. Bail out water. If it doesn't have a built-in shelter, rig up a spray shield and windbreak using any available material.

Dry all wet clothing. If there is no dry clothing, squeeze out as much water as possible and put it back on. Maintain body heat by wrapping up in any available material, e.g., parachute or canvas. If in a group, huddle together. To keep circulation going, do mild exercises but do not disturb the balance of the raft.

In a hot climate: Keep covered in strong sun. Cover head and neck to avoid sunstroke. Protect eyes from glare (see p. 45). Damp down clothes to cool the body, but make sure you are dry by evening, for nights can be very cold and darkness comes quickly in the tropics. Prolonged contact with seawater causes sores.

Air expands with heat, so if it is very hot let some air out of an inflatable. Reinflate in the evening cool.

TRAVELING

If an SOS has been sent, or you are in or near regular shipping lanes, stay in the same vicinity for 72 hours. If none of these circumstances hold, get under way at once to take advantage of initial energy. Assess the nearest shipping lane and head in that direction. Your craft will move with the wind and current—seldom more than 9–13 km (6–8 miles) per day. Take in the sea anchor. Use a paddle as a rudder. If the wind is against your chosen direction stream sea anchor to maintain position.

Take these factors into consideration in making your decision whether to stay or travel:
Has an SOS been sent? Is your position known to rescuers? Do you know it? Is the weather favorable for a search? Are other vessels likely to pass you? How many days supply of food and water have you?

To use the wind: Inflate dinghy fully and sit high. Improvise a sail if necessary. Do not secure its lower edges. Hold lower lines or bottom of sail, then release them in sudden gusts of wind so the raft is not capsized.

In rough water: Stream sea anchor out from the bow to keep it into the wind and prevent capsizing. Keep low. Do not sit on the sides, stand up, or make sudden movements. Tie several rafts or dinghies together.

Assign lookouts, even in darkness, to watch for shipping, aircraft, signs of land, seaweed, fish, birds and flotsam. They should also inspect the raft for signs of leakage or chafing. Watches should be kept short to avoid exhaustion and lack of concentration.

INDICATORS OF LAND NEARBY

Cumulus clouds in an otherwise clear sky are likely to have formed over land. In tropical waters the reflection of sunlight from shallow water over coral reefs produces a green tint on the underside of clouds.

Lone birds may have been blown off course by rough weather, but few seabirds sleep on the water or fly more than 100 miles from land. Their direction of flight is usually outward from land before noon and return in the late afternoon. The continuous sound of bird cries is usually an indication that land is not far away.

Drifting vegetation, e.g., coconuts, may be a sign of land (but they can be carried right across an ocean).

A change in the sea's direction may be caused by the tide pattern around an island. A constant wind with a decreasing swell suggests land to windward.

Water that is muddy with silt is likely to have come from the mouth of a large river.

SIGNALING AT SEA

Use flares, dye markers and movement of any kind to attract attention at sea.

If you have no signaling equipment, wave clothing or tarpaulins and churn the water if it is still. At night or in fog use a whistle to maintain contact with other survivors.

If a radio transmitter is part of the equipment aboard a life raft, instructions for its operation will be found on its side (see p. 209).

Sea markers which release dye are only of use in daytime. They are usually conspicuous for three hours.

Pyrotechnic equipment must be kept secure and dry. Read instructions and beware of fire hazards. When firing flares do not point them downward or toward yourself or anyone else. Use flares only when certain they will be seen. Fire when a plane is flying toward you, not when it has gone past (see pp. 219–220).

HEALTH

Exposure and severe hydration are major problems.

Constipation, difficulty in urinating or concentrated urine are not unusual. Do not attempt to treat them or you could force further liquid loss.

If feeling sick, try not to vomit. Never induce vomiting.

Continued exposure to saltwater can cause boils. Do not prick or squeeze. Do not damp yourself down too often with saltwater. Stop damping yourself with seawater if there is any soreness.

Protect eyes from glare. If eyes are sore moisten a cloth with seawater and place over the eyes and rest them. Do not do this for long, it can make skin sore.

Trenchfoot (see p. 263) can occur when awash with water. Exercise will help protect you from it and from frostbite and exposure. Keep well covered when resting and, when on watch, gently exercise the limbs.

WATER

Even if you have a good water supply, ration it at once. Do not relax the ration until final rescue or until you can replenish it, for you have no idea how long you will have to last out.

WATER RATIONS

Day 1: No water. The body is a reservoir.

Days 2–4: 400 cc (14 oz) if available.

Day 5 onward: 55-225 cc (2-8 oz) daily, depending on climate and water available.

When drinking, moisten lips, tongue and throat before swallowing. Sip slowly—gulping will make you vomit.

Reducing water needs: Reduce sweating. Make use of breezes and seawater to cool the body. If it is very hot and the waters are safe, take a dip over the side—but first check your safety line. You should always be tied on. Beware of dangerous fish and be sure that you can get back aboard.

Take anti-sickness pills, if available, as soon as you feel queasy, for vomiting will lose valuable fluids.

If you are low on water do not eat (see p. 15).

Gathering fresh water: Collect rainwater night and day—rig up a catchment from canvas or plastic. At night rig canvas with edges folded to catch dew. Stow as much in containers as you can. Drink up puddles in the boat first. But be careful in heavy seas as the water will be contaminated with salt.

Sea ice can produce drinking water (see p. 20). In summer, pools on old sea ice may be drinkable (if they are not wave splashes). Taste carefully before drinking.

You can also get water from fish (see p. 22).

Treatment of seawater: Life-raft equipment may include solar stills and desalination kits (see p. 18). Set solar stills out immediately, but use desalination tablets only when the weather is unfavorable for the stills and dew or rain catchment is ineffective.

DO NOT drink seawater
DO NOT drink urine
DO NOT drink alcohol
DO NOT smoke
DO NOT eat, unless water is available

Sleep and rest are the best way of enduring periods of reduced water and food—but make sure that you have adequate shade during the day. If the sea is rough, tie yourself to the raft, close any cover and ride out the storm as best you can. Try to relax.

FOOD

Conserve emergency food supplies until needed. Try to live off sea life. There are dangerous fish but in the open sea, fish are generally safe to eat. Near the shore there are dangerous and poisonous species.

FISHING

Never wrap fishing line around bare hands or tie it to an inflatable dinghy. Salt gives it a sharp cutting edge.

Wear gloves if available or use a cloth to handle fish to avoid injury from sharp fins and gill covers.

Fish and turtles attracted to the shelter provided by a dinghy will swim under it. Pass a net under the keel from end to end (it takes two to hold the ends).

Improvise hooks (see p. 93). If using a metal spoon or spinner keep it moving by paying out and reeling in. Let the "bait" sink and then retrieve it.

Fish flesh spoils easily and must be eaten fresh unless the air is dry when it can be dried in the sun for future meals. Clean and gut before drying.

Birds: Will be attracted to a raft as a potential perching place. Keep still until they settle and try to grab them.

Wrap a diamond-shaped tin gorge with fish and trail to attract birds. When seized by a bird the gorge should lodge across its gullet.

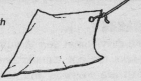

Seaweed: Occurs on shorelines and in floating forms. Raw seaweeds are tough and salty and hard to digest. They absorb fluids—do not eat when water is scarce.

Seaweeds also provide food in the form of small fish, crabs and shrimps living on them. These decapods are not easy to see, being mottled brown, like seaweed.

Make a grapple hook by lashing pieces of wood or metal wreckage together to form a multiple hook. Attach it to a line and trail it, or throw it out to rake in weed. Use it for gathering drifting wreckage to consolidate a raft.

DANGEROUS FISH

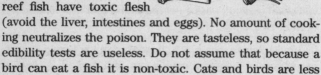

Poisonous fish: Many reef fish have toxic flesh (avoid the liver, intestines and eggs). No amount of cooking neutralizes the poison. They are tasteless, so standard edibility tests are useless. Do not assume that because a bird can eat a fish it is non-toxic. Cats and birds are less susceptible to the toxins than human beings.

Symptoms of poisoning include numbness of the lips, tongue, extremities, severe itching and a reversal of temperature sensations: cold things seem hot and hot things cold. Nausea, vomiting, loss of speech, dizziness and paralysis may follow. They can be fatal.

Aggressive fish: These include the barracuda, which charges at lights or shiny objects at night; the huge sea bass; and the moray eel. Sea snakes are venomous.

SHARKS

The survivor at sea is vulnerable to shark attack. Ocean sharks are not usually ferocious when food is plentiful. Most are cowards and can be scared off by the jab of a stick, especially on the nose. However, making a commotion may attract sharks.

Sharks feed off the ocean bottom, but hungry sharks will follow fish to the surface and into shallow water; their hunger at such times makes them dangerous.

Sharks feed at night, dusk and dawn, locating prey by smell and vibration. They seek easy prey (wounded fish and stragglers) and are attracted by blood, bodily wastes and rubbish (they will scavenge refuse thrown overboard).

Weak movements draw attention. Strong, regular movements and loud noises repel them. Human appearance is strange to a shark and clothing produces a confusing shape. A group of clothed humans bunched together will be safer than a lone individual. If a shark keeps its distance, it is only curious. If it circles inward and makes sudden movements, attack is likely.

PROTECTION AGAINST SHARKS: IN THE WATER

Avoid passing body wastes. If you must urinate do it in short spurts and allow it to dissipate between spurts. Collect feces and throw far away. Try to hold vomit in the mouth and reswallow it (or throw it far away). If you must swim use strong strokes; avoid schools of fish.

Sharks cannot stop or turn quickly. A good swimmer can evade a single shark by rapid changes of direction.

If in a group, bunch together and face outward. Kick and punch out with a stiff arm using heel of hand. Slap the water with cupped hands. Put your head under and shout. If you have a knife, let the shark take it in the snout, or go for the gills and eyes.

PROTECTION AGAINST SHARKS: ON A BOAT

Don't fish when sharks are around. Don't throw waste overboard. Let go of baited hooks. Do not trail arms or legs in the water. To deter a shark from attacking, jab its snout with a paddle or pole. Beware: a large shark could take a bite out of a boat.

If you catch a small shark, haul it to the side of the craft, pull the head clear, and club hard before approaching and finishing it off with more blows. Don't try this with a large shark. It could injure you and your craft. Cut your line and sacrifice part of it—the shark's threshing will soon attract its fellows.

MAKING A LANDFALL

When approaching land, select a landing point where it will be easy to beach or swim ashore. Take down the sail; the sea anchor will keep you pointing at the shore and will slow down your progress. Steer away from rocks. Try not to land with the sun in your eyes.

A sloping beach with a small surf is ideal. Try to ride the back of a breaker. To avoid being swamped by an oncoming wave paddle hard, but do not overshoot a breaker which is carrying you along. In heavy surf point vessel seaward and paddle into an approaching wave.

Note the lie of the land: high ground, vegetation, watercourses. If with companions, choose a rendezvous point in case you are separated. Do not try to land at night—it is too dangerous. Wait until morning.

If you float into an estuary try to reach a bank. The turning tide could carry you back out to sea. Take in the sea anchor and make the boat as light as possible. Bail out an inflatable and inflate it to the maximum to make the most of the incoming tide. If being swept back out to sea by the ebb, ballast the dinghy by part-filling it with water and stream the sea anchor.

> **Tie yourself to the raft. Even if it is overturned or damaged and you are rendered unconscious, you stand a chance of surviving, whereas alone in the water and dashed on the rocks—you will be killed.**

If swimming ashore in a heavy sea, keep on clothing, shoes and life jacket. Raise legs, knees bent, and take the shock of impact of the rocks on the soles of your feet.

RESCUE

THE first requirement for rescue is to let others know of your situation and your location. Once contact has been made you can pass on other information.

SIGNALING

SOS (Save Our Souls) is an internationally recognized distress signal. Mayday (from *m'aidez*: French for *help me*) is the signal used in radio-telecommunications.

Almost any signal repeated three times will serve as a distress signal: three fires, or columns of smoke; three whistles, or shots, or flashes of light. If using noises or lights, wait one minute between each group of three.

Transmitters: Dinghies, life rafts and jackets are often equipped with transmitters which indicate position over a short range. To avoid wasting precious batteries, hold in reserve until there is a chance of their signals being picked up. With long-range transmitters, send distress signals at regular intervals. Frequencies are usually preset at 121.5 and 243 megacycles and the range is about 32 km (20 miles). Portable VHF transceivers can communicate only with stations in a direct line of sight and without any intervening obstruction (though a relay station may be established on a high point). Such sets are usually tuned to a mountain rescue frequency but procedures should be established before departure.

If you have a transmitter, check the batteries. Can an engine be used to generate electricity or recharge the batteries? Conserve fuel and plan your transmissions to a pattern rather than attempting long periods on air.

The International Mountain Distress Signal is six whistles a minute (or six waves, light flashes, etc.) followed by a minute's silence, then repeated.

Siting signals

Take account of the terrain. Choose high points for light signals. Erect an unusual silhouette on a ridge to attract attention.

Planes fly over hilly territory from the lower to the higher ridges. Thus slopes behind ridges may be hidden as the plane approaches. Signals near tops of ridges should be seen from any direction. Lay out marks on level ground or on slopes that are not likely to be overlooked.

Vehicle or aircraft wreckage: A stranded vehicle or downed aircraft provides useful signaling aids. Fuel, oil and hydraulic fluid can be burned. Tires and electrical insulation generate smoke. Glass and chrome make good reflectors. Life jackets, dinghies, and parachutes are eye-catching. Arrange colorful, shiny objects in a visible spot to attract attention to your location.

Switch lights on at night. If batteries are low, keep them in reserve to flash headlamps and sound the horn.

Fire and smoke: Establish signal fires once immediate needs for treatment of injury and provision of shelter have been met. Gather fuel for camp and signal fires.

Place three fires in a triangle at equal distances apart. Failing that, a group of clearly separated fires will serve. If fuel is scarce, use only your campfire.

Signal fires should be kept dry, and maintained, ready to be lit to attract attention of passing aircraft. Use tinder to get them going rapidly (see p. 119).

Gasoline can be used as a firelighter but don't just pour it on. Lay a piece of gasoline-soaked rag among the tinder. Don't light it at once. Carry the fuel can off to a safe distance. Wait a few seconds, then light the wick. If a fire does not light the first time pull tinder apart and check for sparks or embers, before adding extra gasoline.

> Keep a stock of green boughs, oil or rubber close by to create smoke if needed. Among vegetation or close to trees, build an earth wall around each fire to contain it. Do not build fires among trees where the canopy will block out the signal. Place them in a clearing.

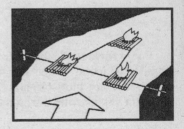

If by a lake or river, build rafts to place your fires on and anchor or tether them securely in position. Arrow indicates direction of current.

Torch trees: Use small, isolated trees for fire signals. Build a fire between the boughs using dry twigs or old bird's nests. This will ignite the foliage, producing lots of smoke. Fires at the base of dead trees burn for a long time, but don't risk starting a forest fire. Apart from the damage this will cause, your life will be in jeopardy.

Luminous cone fires: On a clear, open site make a tripod with a platform to support a fire. Use evergreen boughs as cover to keep the cone dry; they will burn brightly and give off smoke. Cover the entire cone with bright-colored material, e.g., a parachute, which will itself be noticeable by day. Whip it off when you ignite the fire—you may not attract attention the first time.

Keep tripods well maintained, ensuring wood is dry. Drive pole ends into ground to prevent tipping in strong winds. A flaming cone fire is visible for miles. In exposed locations make a tepee of fabric with smoke and heat outlet at top to keep fire under control. Add fuel from side so as not to mask firelight.

Use wreckage to help fire signaling: Stand a fire on a piece of metal. When hot it increases convection and makes the fire burn brightly. If polished, it will act as a reflector, intensifying the brightness.

SMOKE INDICATORS

By day smoke is a good locator. Have a supply of smoke-producing material ready to put on your fires. Smoke not only helps rescue aircraft find you, it also shows surface wind direction. Make sure smoke is downwind of landing site and of any panel codes you have laid so it does not obscure them from above.

Light smoke stands out against dark earth or forest. Use green grass, leaves, moss and ferns. Wet materials produce a good smudge fire, e.g., damp seat covers smolder for a long time. The smoke also keeps insects at bay.

Dark smoke shows best against snow or desert sand. Use rubber or oil to produce it. If atmospheric conditions make the smoke hang in layers along the ground, build up the fire to increase its height. Thermal currents will then take the smoke to a good height.

Be imaginative: On a river a noticeable floating object carrying a message may attract attention, e.g., a small raft with a bright sail labeled SOS for instance.

If rescue is unlikely and you start making your own way back, leave clear signs so that searchers have an indication of the route you have taken. Stay close to regular flight routes or keep to open territory.

CODES

GROUND-TO-AIR SIGNALING

Attract attention during daylight, even if you are asleep or injured with the following signals. Make them as large and as noticeable as possible. A recommended size is 10 m long and 3 m wide (40 ft x 10 ft) for each symbol, with 3 m (10 ft) between symbols.

Lay panel codes in the open; avoid steep gullies or ravines and do not make them on reverse slopes. Use the marker panels from your survival pouch (see p. 10), or improvise. Lay out wreckage or dig a shallow trench: banked up earth increases the depth of the shadow. Use rocks or boughs to accentuate it. On snow, trampled-out symbols will show clearly until the next snowfall.

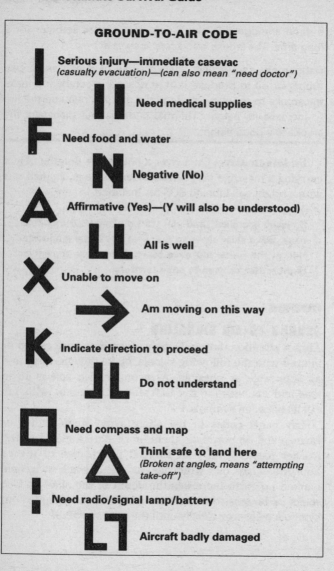

GROUND-TO-AIR CODE

I Serious injury—immediate casevac
(casualty evacuation)—(can also mean "need doctor")

II Need medical supplies

F Need food and water

N Negative (No)

A Affirmative (Yes)—(Y will also be understood)

LL All is well

X Unable to move on

→ Am moving on this way

K Indicate direction to proceed

JL Do not understand

□ Need compass and map

△ Think safe to land here
(Broken at angles, means "attempting take-off")

: Need radio/signal lamp/battery

L7 Aircraft badly damaged

Once contact has been made, a message signaled by the aircraft can be answered with A or Y (affirmative) and N (negative) signals, or Morse code or body signals.

Night signals: Use inflammable substances to make signals which will work at night. Dig or scrape an SOS (or any symbol) in the earth, sand or snow and, when the signal is needed, pour gasoline into it and ignite it.

Message signaling

International Morse code can be transmitted by flashing lights on and off, by a heliograph, by waving a flag or a shirt tied to a stick. Always carry a copy of the code.

Heliograph: Use the sun and a reflector to flash light signals. Any shiny object will do—polished tin, glass, a piece of foil—but a hand mirror is best. Long flashes are dashes and quick ones dots. If you do not know Morse code, random flashes should attract attention. At least learn the code for SOS. A flash can be seen at a great distance and requires little energy. Sweep the horizon during the day. If a plane approaches make intermittent flashes or you may dazzle the pilot. Once you have been seen, stop signaling.

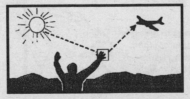

With an improvised single-sided reflector pick up sunlight to get an image on the ground or some other surface and lead it in the direction of the aircraft.

Punch a hole in a double-sided reflector to improvise a heliograph. Sight target you wish to contact through hole in heliograph (a) in the direction of the sun, so sun shines through hole (b). You will see a spot of light on your face (c). Angle mirror so dot of light on your face "disappears" back through hole in mirror—still sighting your contact.

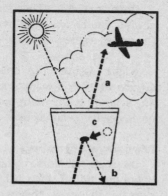

If your attempts are unsuccessful, bring the mirror close to your eyes with a hand lined up between you and the contact. Angle the mirror to flash on to your hand, then move hand away.

Practice this form of signaling, but unless in a survival situation, do not signal to aircraft or transmit messages which could cause alarm or danger to others.

Rag signals: Tie a flag or a piece of bright-colored clothing to a pole. Move it left for dashes and right for dots. Exaggerate with a figure-of-eight movement.

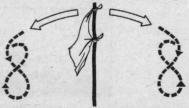

For a "dot" swing to the right and make a figure-of-eight; for a "dash" swing to the left and make a figure-of-eight.

At close range, this may work without figure-of-eight movements. Keep "dash" pauses on the left, slightly longer than "dot" movements to the right.

MORSE CODE

A	.-	N	-.	1	.----
B	-...	O	---	2	..---
C	-.-.	P	.--.	3	...--
D	-..	Q	--.-	4	...-
E	.	R	.-.	5	.....
F	..-.	S	...	6	-....
G	--.	T	-	7	--...
H	....	U	..-	8	---..
I	..	V	...-	9	----.
J	.---	W	.--	0	-----
K	-.-	X	-..-		
L	.-..	Y	-.--		
M	--	Z	--..		

SENDING SIGNALS   (* Send as one word. No pauses)

AAAAA* etc.—Call sign. I have a message

AAA*—End of sentence. More follows

Pause—End of word. More follows

EEEEE* etc.—Error. Start from last correct word

AR—End of message

RECEIVING SIGNALS

TTTTT* etc. I am receiving you

K—I am ready. Start message

T—Word received

IMI*—Repeat sign. I do not understand

R—Message received

USEFUL WORDS

SOS	...---...
SEND	...I.I-.I-..
DOCTOR	-..I---I-.-.I-I---I.-.
HELP	....I.I.-..I.--.
INJURY	..I-.I.---I..-.I-.I-.--
TRAPPED	-I.-.I.-.I.--.I.--.I.I-..
LOST	.-..I---I...I-
WATER	.--I.-I-I.I.-.

BODY SIGNALS

Use these to signal to airmen. Make all signals in a clear and exaggerated manner. Note changes from frontal to sideways positions and use of leg and body posture as well as hand movements. Use a cloth in the hand to emphasize YES and NO signals.

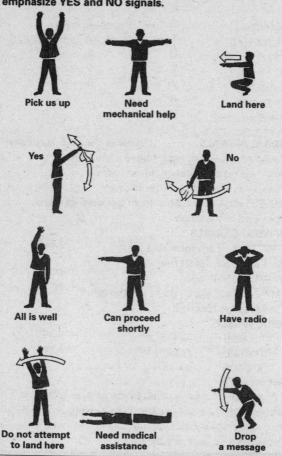

Pick us up

Need
mechanical help

Land here

Yes

No

All is well

Can proceed
shortly

Have radio

Do not attempt
to land here

Need medical
assistance

Drop
a message

Pilots will respond to body signals as follows:

Message received and understood
In daylight: tipping the plane's wings from side to side
At night: flashing green lights

Message received but not understood
In daylight: flying the plane in a right-handed circle
At night: flashing red lights

Mountain rescue code
* Repeat after 1 minute interval
Message: SOS
Flare signal: Red
Sound signal: 3 short blasts, 3 long, 3 short*
Light signal: 3 short flashes, 3 long, 3 short*
Message: HELP NEEDED
Flare signal: Red
Sound signal: 6 blasts in quick succession*
Light signal: 6 flashes in quick succession*
Message: MESSAGE UNDERSTOOD
Flare signal: White
Sound signal: 3 flashes in quick succession*
Light signal: 3 flashes in quick succession*
Message: RETURN TO BASE
Flare signal: Green
Sound signal: Prolonged succession of blasts
Light signal: Prolonged succession of flashes

Flares
Any flare will be investigated in a search, but choose one best fitted to the location. In closely wooded country green does not stand out but red does. Over snow, white merges—green and red are best.

Make sure you understand the instructions, as some

flares eject a white-hot ball of magnesium that will burn a hole in anything it hits—your chest or dinghy.

Some flares are hand-held and reversible. One end produces smoke for daytime, the other a flare for night. The higher these are held the easier they are to see. Flares fired into the air can be seen from afar.

Keep flares dry and away from naked flames and heat sources. Ensure safety pins are in position and secure, but may be easily removed when necessary.

Handling flares: Hand-held flares are cylindrical tubes with a cap at each end. The top cap is often embossed so it can be identified by touch. Remove it first. Then remove base cap, exposing a short string and safety pin, or other safety device. Point flare upward and away from you and anyone else. Remove pin, or turn to the fire position. Hold flare at arm's length, shoulder-height, pointing up. Tug the firing string vertically downward. Brace yourself for the kickback. Some flares have a spring-mechanism trigger.

To fire Very pistols, load, point skyward, cock the hammer and squeeze the trigger. Mini-flares are lighter than Very pistols but as effective. Handle with care. To use, screw a flare of the selected color into the end of the discharger, aim skyward, pull back striker and fire!

> ☠ Hand-held flares get hot. When they burn down do not drop them into the bottom of a boat, where they could start a fire or burn straight through an inflatable.

INFORMATION SIGNALS

If you abandon camp leave clear direction markers to indicate your route. Continue to make them, not only for people to follow but to establish your own route as a guide if you start going back on your trail.

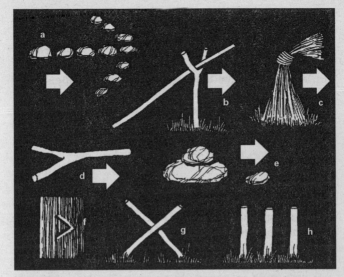

Place rocks or debris in arrow shape (a) to be visible from the air. Ground level signs include: stick in crooked support, with the top indicating direction followed (b); grasses tied in an overhand knot with end hanging in direction followed (c); forked branches laid with fork pointing in direction followed (d); small rocks on larger rocks, with small rock beside (e), indicating a turn or arrow notches cut in tree trunks (f). A cross of sticks or stones (g) means "not this way." Signal danger or emergency with 3 rocks, sticks or clumps of grass.

SEARCH

A search will start from the last known location and sweep on the proposed route. An assessment will be made of probable strategy adopted. The search will then be extended to cover the whole area. Ideally this will be done from the air but severe weather may mean it has to be done on foot.

Aerial search patterns will cover both sides of the intended flight path of missing aircraft or your known route. If weather conditions permit, a night search will be made, for lights will be visible from a great height and a wider area can thus be covered.

If you are signaling to an aircraft and it turns away, keep watching. It may be following a search pattern and you will be able to anticipate when to signal again.

Most aerial searches involve parallel sweeps toward and away from the sun so any reflection from a missing aircraft or other wreckage and signals will be seen.

At sea, combined sea-and-air searches allow aircraft to locate survivors so that ships can pick them up.

HELICOPTER RESCUE

Helicopters are frequently used to carry out rescues. Where possible the pilot will land to take on survivors and fly them out. Survivors should check out suitable landing sites and create a site if necessary.

A helicopter requires an obstruction-free approach and exit path, both into prevailing winds. The ground should be level—a slope of no more than 7° (a gradient of 1 in 10) is acceptable. The touchdown surface must be firm and free of loose materials—no leaves, etc.

SELECTING AND PREPARING A LANDING SITE

Find a natural clearing at least 26 m (80 ft) in diameter. A further 5 m (15 ft) should be cleared to a height of 60 cm (2 ft). It must have a clear approach path into the prevailing wind with no obstructions within an angle of 15° of the landing pad (LP). In close country, seek a riverbank on a large bend. On level high ground, fell trees so they fall downhill, clear of approach and exit paths. Don't attempt to cut an LP on flat ground.

Mark touchdown point with an H made of rocks (keep surface smooth), or securely anchored clothing. Stamp snow down firmly to stop it swirling. Water dry surfaces to keep dust down. In mountains updrafts and downdrafts can be considerable. Select a site giving maximum lift in take-off direction.

Use smoke to indicate direction and strength of wind, but make sure it doesn't obscure the touchdown area. If a fire is not practical make a T sign from contrasting material and place it at downwind edge of LP with horizontal bar of T placed upwind. Or stand on far downwind side of the LP with arms outstretched and back to the wind to signal. Don't do this too soon, and then only in the correct position. It is similar to the body signal "need help."

For a night rescue use flares and fires to indicate your position. If using torches or other beams, shine them skyward to attract attention, then shine them on to the touchdown or winching area. Don't dazzle the pilot.

When helicopter touches down, do not approach from the rear. This is a blind spot for the crew and the tail rotor is unprotected. On sloping ground always approach up the slope, never down a slope.

Do not carry anything which could foul the main rotor. Keep sharp objects away from body panels of 'copter. Sit in the seat allocated to you by the crewman, fasten the seat belt and keep fastened until told otherwise. Do not try to alight until engine has been shut down after you have landed—even then, wait for directions.

Non-landing rescue: If an LP is impossible you can be winched up while the helicopter hovers.

If survivors are being lifted from a ship place deck at 40° to the right of the eye of the wind. Try to give a wind speed over the deck of about 29 kph (18 mph).

WINCHING TECHNIQUES

Double lift: A crewman is lowered on the winch with another strop for the survivor. During the lift, crewman supports survivor with his legs and hands. After the strop has been put in place and tightened keep your arms down by sides and do not lift them.

Single lift: Fit yourself into the strop. When you have placed it under your armpits and securely tightened the grommet give the "thumbs up" sign. Make no further signals until on board. When you reach the cabin doorway, do exactly as winchman directs.

If on a raft, disconnect yourself from lifeline. Fold down cover and lower sails. Stream the sea anchor to assist the pilot in trapping raft under rotor downwash.

Aircraft build up static electricity. This is discharged when the aircraft, or the cable, touches the ground. Allow winch sling or cable to touch down before you approach it, or you will get a substantial electric shock.

HEALTH

TAKE precautions to avoid illness and injury, but make sure that in the event medical problems do arise everyone in the group knows first aid. If there is no hope of expert help, the survivor may have to take drastic measures to save a life. Some of the advice given in this section is intended only for such circumstances.

FIRST AID

PRIORITIES

Where there are many casualties, treat those with multiple injuries, bleeding, breathing and heart trouble first. Assess injuries and handle in this sequence:

1 **Restore and maintain breathing/heartbeat**
2 **Stop bleeding**
3 **Protect wounds and burns**
4 **Immobilize fractures**
5 **Treat shock**

 The possibility of AIDS infection demands care in dealing with blood and wounds. Cover your hands with gloves or plastic bags.

REDUCING DANGER

Before approaching a casualty, check for danger from falling debris, gas, traffic, etc. Switch current off before touching electrocution victims (see p. 230).

If possible, examine patient before moving, but if there is danger move patient to safety. Those with spinal injuries are at risk when moved (see p. 249).

UNCONSCIOUS CASUALTIES

Check whether they are breathing and begin artificial respiration immediately if necessary. Check for external bleeding and injury. Establish cause of unconsciousness.

Unconscious but breathing

Check there is no spinal injury, clear obstructions in the mouth, deal with any serious bleeding and place them in recovery position. Turn patient on one side (by grasping clothing at hip). Loosen tight clothing.

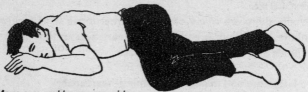

Move arm and leg on one side outward to stop patient lying flat.
Bend elbow and knee. Turn head in same direction. Lay other arm along other side of patient. Allow other leg to bend slightly to produce a stable position. Check airway is clear.

Do not place a casualty with a suspected spinal injury in the recovery position. Use an artificial airway if available to maintain respiration.

BREATHING AND PULSE

Loud breathing, froth around nose or lips, blueness of lips and ears all indicate difficulty breathing. Check breathing regularly: listen near the nose and mouth. Remove obstructions. If breathing stops, give artificial respiration (see p. 230).

Check at neck or wrist for pulse (see p. 233).

CESSATION OF BREATHING

This dire emergency may be caused by:

Choking, or blockage of air passages (see below)

Drowning or electric shock (see pp. 229–230)

Inhalation of smoke, gases or flame (see p. 229)

Lack of oxygen (see p. 229)

Compression of the chest (see p. 229)

CHOKING AND BLOCKAGES

If breathing has stopped, remove any obstruction in the airway, sweep mouth with a finger and ensure tongue has not fallen back. Give artificial respiration.

If a person can inhale and cough, encourage them to cough out blockage. If they cannot clear the airway, use the Heimlich maneuver with adults (see p. 228 for methods to use on infants and other special cases).

Heimlich maneuver:

Stand behind a conscious casualty, arms around them. Make a fist of one hand and press it thumb inward above navel but below breastbone. Clasp other hand around the fist. Pull sharply upward and inward four times.

If this does not work, give 4 sharp blows to the back between shoulderblades and repeat the maneuver. Check to see if the blockage is dislodged. Repeat—do not give up.

Place unconscious casualty on his or her back, head tilted back. Kneel astride or alongside, place your hands, one on top of the other, with heels of your hands resting above navel. Keep fingers clear. With arm straight, make quick thrusts upward and inward as if to center of ribcage. Thrusts must be strong enough to dislodge blockage. If

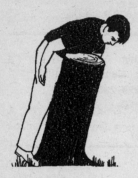

unsuccessful, roll patient on to side and strike four times between shoulder blades. Repeat abdominal thrust as necessary.

Self-help
If alone, use Heimlich maneuver by pulling or pushing against a blunt projection (e.g., a tree or a chair back).

CHOKING: SPECIAL CASES

Children: Hold upside down by heels and strike 4 blows with heel of your hand between the shoulder blades. Alternatively, lay child over your lap, head down, supporting child under chest. Slap back with heel of hand. If blockage is not dislodged, apply Heimlich maneuver with one hand. Use less pressure than for an adult, but it must be sufficient to clear blockage.

Babies: Use much less pressure for back slaps. If blockage is not dislodged, put 2 fingers of one or both hands between navel and bottom of breastbone. Press down and forward quickly, repeat 4 times.

Pregnant women: Position fists against middle of breastbone and thrust upward and inward.

PREVENTING ASPHYXIATION

Pressure on chest can cause asphyxiation. In an avalanche or landslide, crouch with arms bent and elbows tucked well in to protect the chest. A climber who slips and is suspended by a rope around his chest will find it hard to breathe. Pass down a loop (see p. 155) to relieve the pressure.

If wreckage cannot be lifted off a trapped person, use a lever to raise it and prop securely.

Smoke and gas can be prevented entering lungs by placing a fine mesh over nose and mouth. Casualties must have fresh air. Get upwind or use a respirator.

Lack of oxygen is a danger in shelters with no ventilation. A fire adds the risk of carbon monoxide poisoning. Casualties must have fresh air.

Carbon monoxide poisoning is deadly in confined spaces, but is hard to detect. Symptoms resemble alcohol overdose: impaired memory and judgment, and a disregard of danger.

Insure adequate ventilation when using stoves. To test whether there is sufficient oxygen, light a candle: if the flame gets longer and higher, there is a severe lack of oxygen: ventilate. Casualties must have fresh air.

NOT BREATHING/NO PULSE

DROWNING

Symptoms: Can occur through fluid blockages, but patient is often immersed. Face, especially lips and ears, livid and congested; fine froth at mouth, nostrils.

Treatment: Do not attempt to remove liquid from lungs. Begin artificial respiration (see p. 230) as soon as possible. If still in water, support body and begin mouth-to-mouth after removing any obstructions.

ELECTROCUTION

SYMPTOMS: Heart may stop; muscle spasms may throw victim some distance. Electrical burns will be much deeper than they appear.

Treatment: Do not touch until current is off. It may be possible to break contact by pulling on insulated cable to disengage. But beware—liquids will conduct current (victims may urinate). Give artificial respiration and treat for cardiac arrest (see p. 234), then treat burns.

LIGHTNING

Symptoms: Victim usually stunned, or unconscious. Clothing may catch fire. Electrical burns will be most severe where metal objects (jewelry, etc.) are worn.

Treatment: Give artificial respiration (see below) if necessary and treat burns (see pp. 240–241). Prolonged resuscitation may be needed. Recovery often delayed.

POISONING

SYMPTOMS: Poisons which enter lungs or attack the nervous system can cause asphyxia (see p. 255).

HEART ATTACK

SYMPTOMS: Severe chest pain, shortness of breath, giddiness, collapse, anxiety, heavy sweating, irregular pulse, blueness of lips or skin.

Treatment: If breathing fails give artificial respiration and cardiac compression (see p. 234) if pulse stops.

ARTIFICIAL RESPIRATION (AR)

With any form of resuscitation the first five minutes are the most critical, but if breathing does not start, keep artificial respiration up for at least an hour. In a group, take turns. Don't give up!

Mouth-to-mouth ("Kiss of life")

The fastest and most effective method. Begin as soon as airway cleared. If face is injured, or poison or chemical burns are suspect, use Silvester method (see below).

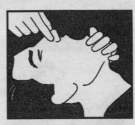

Lie patient on back, tilt head back, hold jaw well open and nostrils closed. Check mouth and throat clear. Loosen tight clothing. Take deep breath, place mouth over patient's mouth and blow.

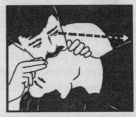

Watch for chest to rise (if it does not, airway may be blocked: treat for choking, see p. 227). Remove your mouth and chest will fall. Repeat quickly 6 times, then continue at a rate of 12–16 inflations a minute until breathing is restored.

For a child: Seal your mouth around the baby's or child's mouth and nostrils. Don't tilt baby's head back too far. Breathe gently into lungs, 20 inflations a minute. Check pulse after two inflations.

> **AIDS: The danger of infection is small, but if you feel at risk, place a clean handkerchief or a thin polythene bag with a small slit in it between your mouth and that of the victim. Blow through the slit or handkerchief.**

Silvester method

Use when poisoning or facial injury prevent mouth-to-mouth, and when patient needs cardiac compression.

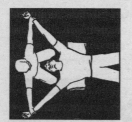

Lie victim on back, raise shoulders with pad of folded material. Kneel astride victim's head, place hands flat over lower ribs and rock forward to press steadily downward.

Lift victim's arms upward and outward as far as possible. Repeat rhythmically 12 times a minute for adults. If there is no improvement, treat for choking to clear blocked airway, then resume artificial respiration treatment.

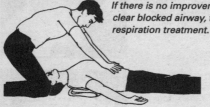

AFTER BREATHING HAS BEEN RESTORED:
Place patient in recovery position—after all forms of resuscitation. But not in cases of spinal injury.

Holger Nielson method

Use to resuscitate a drowning victim if mouth-to-mouth not possible. Facedown position allows liquids to flow freely from mouth without choking the patient.

Lay victim facedown, head turned to one side, arms bent, forehead resting on hands. Loosen tight garments, clear mouth of weed, mud, etc., and insure tongue is brought forward.

Kneel at head, facing casualty. Place your hands over shoulder blades, thumbs touching and fingers spread. Perform the following procedure to a count of eight:

1-2-3 Rock forward with arms straight, producing gentle, even, increasing pressure (about 2 seconds).

4 Rock back, sliding hands to grasp victim's upper arms (½–1 second).

5-6-7 Pull and raise victim's arms gently by rocking farther backward

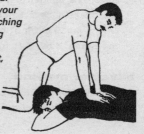

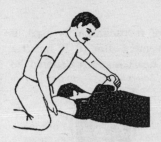

(2 seconds). Avoid raising torso or disturbing head too much.

8 Lower victim's arms to ground and slide hands back to initial position *(½–1 second).*

Repeat 12 times a minute

If victim's arms are injured, place folded garment under forehead and lift under armpits. This is impracticable if ribs or shoulders are badly damaged.

IS HEART BEATING?

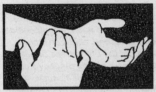

Taking pulse at wrist
Rest fingers lightly at front of wrist, about 1 cm (⅓ in) from thumb side at lower end of forearm.

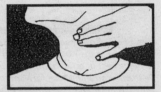

Taking pulse at neck
Turn face to one side. Slide fingers from Adam's apple into groove alongside and press gently.

In a relaxed adult the normal pulse rate is 60–80 beats per minute (average 72); in young children 90–140 per minute. The rate increases with excitement.

Count the beats in 30 seconds and multiply by two. Use a watch with a seconds hand to keep timing accurate; note the result.

If you cannot feel a pulse and the pupils of the eyes are much larger than normal, start cardiac compression while artificial respiration is continued. Mouth-to-mouth and Silvester methods allow both activities to be carried out at same time.

CARDIAC COMPRESSION

Regardless of which method of resuscitation is used, if there is no pulse and no improvement after 10–12 breaths, cardiac compression (external heart massage) should be started.

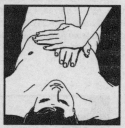

Cardiac compression
Lay casualty on their back on a firm surface and kneel alongside.
Place heel of one hand on lower half of breastbone, about an inch above where the ribs meet, not on the end of the breastbone or below it. Place heel of other hand on top. Keep fingers off the casualty's chest. With arms straight, rock forward and press down about 4 cm (1½ in) 15 times. Repeat about 80 times a minute—more than once per second. Press smoothly and firmly. Erratic or rough pressure could cause injury.

Infants and children: Use less pressure and more compressions. For a baby or toddler, light pressure with two fingers is enough at 100 compressions per minute. Depress chest only 2.5 cm (1 in). For children up to 10 years, use heel of one hand only and push lightly 90–100 times per minute to depth of 3.5 cm (1⅜ in). Give 5 compressions to one lung inflation.

> ☠ **Compression should only be carried out by a trained first aider. Never give compression if the heart is beating—even if only a very faint pulse can be felt. You could stop the heart.**

AR WITH COMPRESSION

If alone, use mouth-to-mouth or Silvester methods of resuscitation, give 2 lung inflations, 15 compressions and repeat. Check for pulse after one minute, and then at 3-minute intervals. Don't give up.

If two first aiders are present, give 5 compressions followed by one deep inflation on upstroke of fifth compression. Repeat. First aider giving inflations should also check pulse and pupils.

As soon as a pulse is detected, stop compressions but continue inflations until the casualty is breathing unaided. Place the victim in recovery position.

SEVERE BLEEDING

An adult has up to 6 liters (11 pints) of circulating blood. Loss of 0.5 liters (1 pint) causes mild faintness, 1 liter (2 pints) causes faintness, increased pulse rate and shallow breathing. 1.5 liters (3 pints) leads to collapse, more than 2.25 liters (4 pints) can be fatal. Immediate steps must be taken to stop the flow of blood. Internal bleeding may not be apparent. If severe, it often leads to shock and can kill.

> When bleeding is coupled with cessation of breathing, treat both at the same time as a double emergency.

Bleeding from veins and capillaries can be stemmed by simple pressure over the bleeding point, with or without a dressing. Pressure must be kept up for at least 5 to 15 minutes to let clotting take effect. Ideally the wound should be covered with a sterile dressing, but preventing blood loss is the priority, so use any clean, non-fluffy cloth. If no dressing is available, use your hand. Squeeze edges of a gaping wound together. If wound is on a limb, raise it above level of heart—lay the victim down and prop up the head or limbs. If you are wounded and alone, use a free hand to apply direct pressure to wound.

> If anything is embedded in the wound, do not try to remove it. Apply pressure beside the fragment.

Arterial bleeding

Speed is vital in stopping blood spurting from an artery. Compress the artery at pressure points where it runs near the surface over a bone. Watch the wound: if blood flow does not lessen, move your fingers until it does. The figures and captions below and overleaf show where to apply pressure to staunch arterial bleeding.

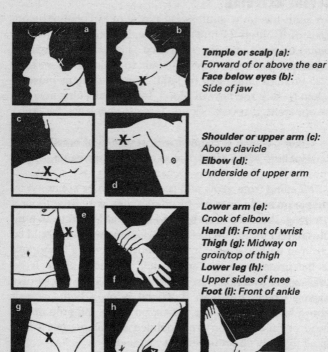

Temple or scalp (a):
Forward of or above the ear
Face below eyes (b):
Side of jaw

Shoulder or upper arm (c):
Above clavicle
Elbow (d):
Underside of upper arm

Lower arm (e):
Crook of elbow
Hand (f): Front of wrist
Thigh (g): Midway on groin/top of thigh
Lower leg (h):
Upper sides of knee
Foot (i): Front of ankle

> Do not apply pressure for more than 15 minutes. You will cut off the blood supply to the tissues.

When bleeding is under control, apply a sterile dressing and bandage securely but not so tight as to cut off circulation. Do not lift the dressing—if a clot is disturbed the bleeding will be made worse.

> After bandaging a limb, check circulation frequently. Loosen a dressing if toes or fingers are blue, cold or numb; risk of gangrene if dressings are too tight. Never use a tourniquet.

Lesser bleeding

Clean the wound carefully and apply a sterile dressing. To avoid risk of infection, do not touch the wound or allow non-sterile materials to touch it. Replace the dressing only when it becomes very dirty.

For a nose bleed, sit the patient up with head slightly forward and pinch soft part of the nostrils for 10 minutes. The patient must breathe through the mouth and not sniff or blow the nose. Loosen tight clothing.

Internal bleeding

This serious condition is common after a violent blow, broken bones or penetrating wounds. Hard to detect.

SYMPTOMS

Victim feels light-headed, restless and faint; looks pale; skin cold, clammy to touch; pulse weak but very fast.

Red/wine-colored urine (injury to kidney/bladder)

Blood passed with feces (lower bowel injury)

Blood vomited (stomach injury)

Blood coughed up as red froth (damage to lungs)

Lie the patient flat with legs slightly elevated. Keep the patient warm but do not overheat. Serious internal bleeding requires expert medical care.

WOUNDS AND DRESSINGS

Open wounds are at risk from infection, especially from tetanus—immunization is essential for adventurers.

Foreign bodies must be extracted with sterile tweezers. Other than in a survival situation, this is best left to trained medics. Cut away clothing, clean the area and irrigate wounds to wash out dirt. Clean wound from center out, do not swab from outside in. Dry and apply a clean dressing. Immobilize wound in a position that is comfortable. Dressings should be changed if they become wet, give off a bad smell, or if pain increases and throbs, indicating infection.

Treat local infection by soaking in hot salty water, or applying poultices to draw out pus. Anything that can be mashed can be used as poultice: rice, potatoes, shredded tree bark, clay. Boil them up and wrap in a cloth. Apply to infected area as hot as can be tolerated. Don't scald. Applied heat, e.g., a warm rock wrapped in cloth, can also aid healing.

Soap is antiseptic: use to wash wounds. Wash hands in boiled water before cleaning wound. Wash wound in boiled water or if none is available use urine, which is sterile and will not introduce infection.

Stitching wounds

Minor wounds, e.g., knife wounds, can be closed by suturing. Clean the wound thoroughly, then stitch across it or use butterfly sutures from your survival kit.

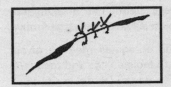

Stitches:
Use sterilized needle and thread or gut. Make each stitch individually, beginning across mid-point of wound. Draw edges together and tie off thread, then work outward.

Adhesive sutures:
Use butterfly sutures or adhesive plasters cut in butterfly shape. Draw edges of wound together. Apply plaster to one side, close up as much as possible and press down on other side.

If the wound becomes infected—red, swollen or tense—remove some or all of stitches to let the pus out. Leave to drain.

Open treatment

The safest way to manage most survival wounds is to cover with a dressing but not suture. If unable to clean thoroughly, the wound must be left to heal from inside.

You may need to drain a deep wound or open an abcess and insert sterilized loose packing of a bandage. Leave a tail hanging out. Allow the wound to drain for a few days. Reduce packing as healing progresses, until able to remove it all and apply a dressing. If lancing or reopening a wound, sterilize the blade first. Do not use antiseptic on deep wounds as there is a risk of tissue damage. Wash the wound with boiled water.

Chest wounds: Place the palm of your hand over sucking wounds (where the chest cavity has been penetrated) to stop air entering. Lay casualty down, head and shoulders supported, inclining to injured side. Plug the wound with large, loose, wet dressing or cover with plastic film or aluminum foil (ideally coated with petroleum jelly) and bandage firmly.

Abdominal wounds: No solids or liquids may be given. Relieve thirst with damp cloth to moisten lips and tongue. If gut is extruded, cover and keep damp. Do not try to push back in place. If no organs extrude, dress and bandage firmly.

Head injuries: Ensure airway is clear and tongue forward. Remove dentures. Control bleeding. Provided there are no spinal injuries, place in recovery position.

Traumatic amputation: Examine wound and tie off exposed arteries with sterile thread.

BURNS

Extinguish burning clothing without fanning the flames. Get the victim down on ground and roll them over, covering with a blanket. Remove smoldering clothes (which retain heat) and tight garments, jewelry, etc.

Reduce the temperature by drenching burned tissues with water to cool them—hold under slow-running cold water for at least 10 minutes. Do not apply antiseptic, butter or ointments. Continue cooling until withdrawal from water does not lead to increase in pain. Leave burns alone except to apply dry, sterile dressing. Put dressings between burned fingers and toes to prevent them sticking to each other. Later, hardwood barks (e.g., oak or beech) can be boiled in water and applied to burned flesh when cool to soothe the wound.

Give the patient plenty of fluids in the form of small cold drinks with a ½ teaspoon of salt or bicarbonate of soda to a pint of water.

Types of burns

Deep burns are charred or white, and bone or muscle may be visible. Superficial burns are much more painful. Blisters should never be burst deliberately. If face and neck are burned, ensure airway is clear. Scalds are caused by liquids—treat as for burns.

Mouth and throat burns are caused by hot gases, hot liquids or corrosive chemicals. Give sips of cold water to cool. Swelling in throat may affect breathing. Give artificial respiration (Silvester method, p. 231) if necessary. With eye burns, hold the lid open and pour plenty of water over the eye to wash out chemicals. Tilt head so the chemical is not washed into mouth or nose.

Use lots of water to dilute or wash off corrosive chemicals and remove clothing. Do not try to neutralize acid with alkali or vice-versa. Treat as for burn. For electrical and lightning burns, see treatment on p. 230. Treat as for heat burns.

> Most burns will result in shock. Flooding extensive burns with cold water may increase shock, but that must be weighed against reducing tissue damage. Keep cooling for at least 10 minutes.

FRACTURES

Examine for broken bones before swelling complicates the task of locating the fracture, and before touching or moving the casualty. Treat urgent injuries such as asphyxia and bleeding first. Immobilize before moving, and finish treatment later.

There are two types of fracture: open (wound open to fracture, or bone pushes through skin) and closed. In open fractures, infection can gain access to bone. If limb is distorted it must be straightened before splinting. It will hurt, so if patient is unconscious do it right away.

SYMPTOMS

Severe pain, aggravated by movement of injured part. Tenderness, even with only gentle pressure. Swelling, with subsequent discoloration or bruising. Deformity: apparent shortening of a limb, irregularity, unnatural movement—compare with unharmed limb. A grating sound when limbs are moved (do not move limbs deliberately to check for this).

If no medical help is expected, reduce closed fractures as soon as possible after injury by applying traction (a slow, strong pull until edges of fractured bone are brought together, then splint and immobilize the whole length of the limb. Splints can be (pieces of wood, rolls of newspaper, ski sticks, etc.) Separate the hard splint material from the skin with padding (moss is ideal) or pressure sores may develop.

If no splint is available, strap the injured limb to the body. Insert padding in natural hollows to keep in position. Secure above and below fracture and below nearest joints. Tie with soft materials, using reef knots. Do not tie splints directly over injury or let knots press against limb. Check the circulation periodically.

Types of fracture
Fracture of arm below elbow, of hand or of fingers:

Place the sling (e.g., long-sleeved sweater) between the arm and body. Immobilize from elbow to mid-fingers with padded splint. Take one arm of shirt behind head. Tie to other on opposite side to injury. Knot below the elbow to prevent slipping. The arm is thus elevated to prevent swelling.

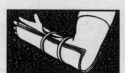
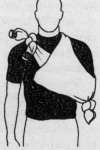

Fracture at the elbow:

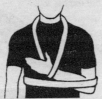

If the elbow is bent, support it in a narrow sling. Bind it across upper arm and chest. Check the pulse to ensure the artery is not trapped. If there is no pulse, straighten the arm a little, and if there is still no pulse, urgent medical aid is required.

If the elbow is straight, do not bend it. Place a pad in the armpit and strap the arm to the body, or place padded splints on either side of arm.

Fracture of the upper arm:
Place a pad in armpit, with a splint from shoulder to elbow on the outside of the arm and a narrow sling at the wrist. Bind the arm.

Fracture of the shoulder blade or collarbone:
Make a sling to take the weight off the injured part, and immobilize it with bandage across the arm and body.

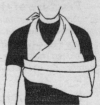

For fractures of the thigh or lower leg, apply a figure-of-eight bandage, binding feet and ankles of both legs.

Fracture of the hip or upper leg:
Place a splint on the inside of the leg and another from ankle to armpit. Use a stick to push tying bands under the hollows of the leg. If no splints are available, pad a folded blanket between the legs and tie the broken leg to the sound leg.

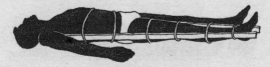

Fracture to the knee:

If the leg is straight, place the splint behind the leg. Apply a cold compress to the knee.

If the leg is bent: bring both legs together, place padding between calves and thighs and strap in those places. This is a temporary measure only. If rescue is unlikely, the leg must be made as straight as possible.

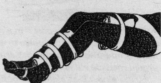

Fracture to the lower leg:

Splint from above the knee to beyond the heel, or pad between the legs and tie them both together (see fracture of the hip or upper leg, p. 243).

Fracture of the ankle or foot:

A splint is not normally used. Elevate the foot to reduce swelling, and immobilize with a folded blanket strapped twice at ankle and once under the foot. If it is a closed fracture, a shoe or boot will provide stability. Do not put weight on the foot.

Fracture of the pelvis:

Symptoms are pain in groin or lower abdomen. Pad between the thighs and tie at the knees and ankles. Place a pillow support below bent legs and strap the patient to a flat support (e.g., a door, stretcher) at shoulder, waist and ankle. Alternatively, place the padding between the legs and bandage around feet, ankles and knees, with two overlapping bandages over the pelvis.

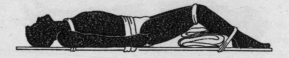

Fracture of the skull: Symptoms include blood or watery fluid seeping from ear or nose. Lay the victim in recovery position, leaking side down. Lightly cover the ear with a sterile dressing, check breathing and pulse. Immobilize.

Fracture of the spine: Symptoms include pain in back and loss of sensation in lower limbs. Ask casualty to move fingers and toes and gently test for feeling. The patient must be immobilized—place soft, solid objects around patient to prevent movement of head or body.

Fracture of the neck:
Immobilization is essential. Use a cervical collar of rolled-up paper or a towel folded to 10–14 cm (4–5½ in) wide to fit from top of breastbone to jaw. Fold the edges to make them narrower at back than front. Overlap around the neck and secure with belt or tie.

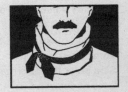

SPRAINS

Tearing of tissues connected to a joint. Symptoms: pain, swelling. Bathe with cold water, support with a bandage (not too tight), elevate limb and rest. Do not put under painful stress or you risk permanent damage. If you must walk on a sprained ankle, keep boot on for support. If in doubt whether a sprain or a break, treat as fracture.

DISLOCATIONS

Symptoms include pain and obvious deformity but no grating sound. Muscle spasms fix bone in position.

Types of dislocation

For a dislocated shoulder, take off your shoe, put your foot in casualty's armpit and pull on the arm.

A dislocated finger should be pulled, then gently released

so bone slips back. Be very gentle with the thumb. If it does not work first time, leave it alone.

If the jaw is dislocated, place a pad of cloth over lower teeth. Rest head on firm support and press down on pads with thumbs, rotating dislocated side of jaw backward and upward. It should snap into place. Bandage around head and under jaw. Feed soft foods.

SHOCK

Shock can kill. Act quickly to prevent it. Symptoms are:

Cold and clammy skin
Casualty weak, dizzy or faint
Shallow and rapid pulse
Casualty may be thirsty
Vomiting or unconsciousness
Skin paler than normal, often grayish
Loss of color in lips

Severe bleeding, loss of body fluids from severe burns or prolonged vomiting or diarrhea commonly lead to shock. Other causes are electrocution and heart attack.

Reassure the casualty and do not excite or move them more than necessary. If they are conscious, lay them flat, legs elevated about 30 cm (1 ft). Loosen tight clothing. The priority is to encourage the supply of blood to the vital organs. Do not give anything to eat or drink. Cover them to keep warm, but do not add heat. Check breathing and pulse, and treat injuries. If there is loss of consciousness, impaired breathing or signs that vomiting may occur, place the casualty in the recovery position.

Stand by to give mouth-to-mouth resuscitation and cardiac compression. Shock can take a long time to pass. Encourage rest and do not move them unnecessarily. If

you appear calm and in control, the patient will feel
cared for and will respond. Never leave a shock victim
on their own.

BANDAGING

A triangular bandage, with short sides not less than 1 m
(or 1 yard) is a versatile dressing for slings and bandages.

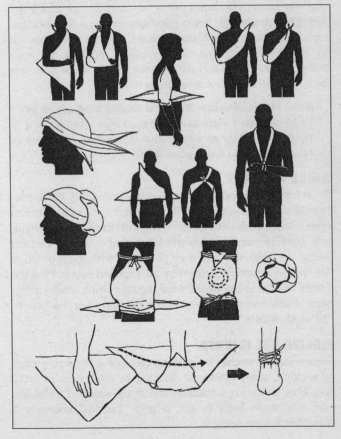

Bandages should be applied firmly enough to stop slipping, but not so tight as to cut into the flesh or interfere with circulation. Crepe bandages are best, but any fabric will do. Keep bandages rolled up; unrolling as you apply helps keep bandages smooth and even.

After applying a dressing (a pad of cotton wool covered with gauze in a sterile wrapping—if you must improvise, use very clean, non-fluffy material—and do not touch the pad when applying), begin bandaging with a firm oblique turn to anchor it. Each turn should overlap previous one by two-thirds, with the edges parallel. Tuck in the ends below the last layer and secure with safety pin or adhesive tape, or tie in reef knot away from wound.

> Never join bandages with knots. Anchor separate strips by binding over a previously applied layer. Tie finishing knots over uninjured side or limb. Use knots which are easily untied and easily accessible.

MINOR AILMENTS

Even minor ailments can turn nasty if untreated. Wash friction blisters, sterilize a needle and pierce the near blister's edge. Gently press out fluid, cover with dressing and bandage. Earache can be relieved by pouring drops of warmed edible oil into the ear and plugging with cotton wool. Toothache is usually caused by an exposed nerve. Plug the cavity with pine-tree resin: scar the tree trunk, soak up the gum which oozes out on cotton wool and plug the hole in the tooth with it.

MOVING THE INJURED

Improvise a stretcher by passing two poles through pieces of sacking, heavy plastic or clothing, or use a door or table top. If no poles are available, roll in the sides of a blanket and use these rolls to get a grip. Test an improvised stretcher before using it.

Loading a stretcher

A patient on a blanket can be lifted using the blanket. Other methods of lifting depend on the number of helpers. Agree signals for synchronized movements.

With 4 persons:

C supports head and shoulders, D hooks fingers with adjoining hands of B and C to aid lift. A, B and C support while D places stretcher in position. D helps lower the patient.

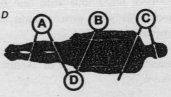

With 3 persons:

Place stretcher at patient's head. C lifts at knees, A and B lock fingers under shoulders and hips. Move casualty from foot of stretcher to over it.

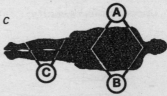

With 2 persons:

Both stand astride casualty. B links arms beneath shoulders, A lifts with one hand under thighs, the other under knees. Both move forward to above stretcher.

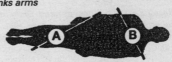

CASUALTIES WITH SPINAL INJURIES

Move only if in danger. Three or four people are needed. Do not bend or twist. One person supports head and neck, another holds shoulders. In absence of stretcher, roll onto blanket. Support head and torso. If working alone do not twist or turn casualty over. Pull by shoulders if facedown, by ankles if faceup, in direction in which body is lying. On rough ground, drag from behind, pulling by shoulders and resting the casualty's head on your forearms.

Lifting on your own

Choose a method you can sustain without dropping the casualty. Lift a light casualty by the cradle method: one arm under thighs, the other under armpit. Alternatively, provided the casualty's arms are not hurt, use the crutch method: place and hold one of their arms around your neck; put your arm around their waist, grasping their clothing at the hip.

The fireman's lift can be used with an unconscious or conscious casualty, but is not suitable if the victim is heavy.

Unconscious casualty:

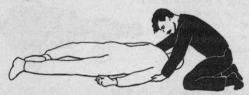

Place face down. Kneel at head. Slide hands under shoulders. Lift under the armpits to a kneeling position, then to upright. Raise their right arm with your left hand. Continue as for conscious casualty (below).

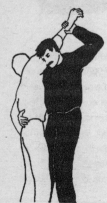

Conscious casualty:
Grasp victim's right wrist. Bend your head under his arm so your shoulder is level with his lower abdomen.

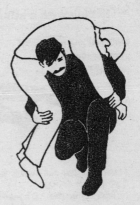

Bend your knees, allowing the weight to fall across your shoulders. Place your right arm between or around legs.

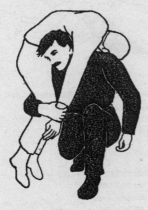

Transfer his right wrist to your right hand and lift, taking weight on your right shoulder.

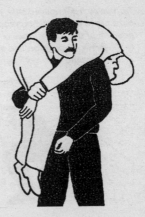

Stand up and adjust the weight across your shoulders. The casualty is head-down—not suitable for facial or head injuries.

Lifting with a sling:

The best one-man-carry
method for long
distances.

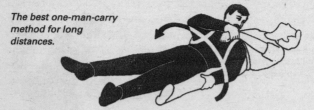

Make a continuous loop to act as
a sling wide enough
not to cut into the
casualty and
long enough to
go over your
shoulders and
twice across
victim's back. Place the sling beneath the victim's thighs and lower back
so two loops protrude. Lie between victim's legs and put your arms
through loops. Tighten the slack. Grasp victim's hand and leg on the
injured side.

Turn away from injured side, rolling so that victim lies on top. Adjust
the sling to make load comfortable and rise to kneeling
position (if the belt is loose or the load insecure, return
to the previous position and adjust). You should be
able to proceed with both hands free.

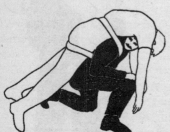

EMERGENCY CHILDBIRTH

Labor can be precipitated by stress. Signs include low backache, regular contractions and discharge of blood-stained mucus. This stage may last several hours; the second stage begins when contractions grow stronger and more frequent. Waters may break at any time. Sterilize scissors or knife and three 20 cm (9 in) lengths of thread. Have plenty of hot water available. Helpers must be healthy (free of colds, infections, or sores) and should scrub hands thoroughly for 4 minutes.

In the second stage, the mother should adopt the most natural position, e.g., a supported squat, but she should not lie down. She should keep her knees drawn up, pulling them up farther as she bears down during contractions. If a bowel movement occurs, wipe clean from front to back. She must stop pushing and pant when baby's head appears. Tear any membrane covering the face. If the umbilical cord is around baby's neck, ease it over the head or loop over shoulder. Support baby's head in palm of your hands; as shoulders appear support body under armpits and lift toward mother's abdomen. Be prepared for baby to be very slippery. Ensuring that no tension is put on the cord, place baby between or by mother's legs, head lower than body. If baby does not appear headfirst and delivery is held up for more than 3 minutes after shoulders emerge, pull very gently.

Clear the baby's mouth with a clean swab. Do not smack. If it does not cry and isn't breathing, begin very gentle mouth-to-mouth resuscitation. When the baby cries, lay it by its mother's breast.

The third stage of labor is delivery of the placenta (10–30 minutes after birth). When it is expelled and cord has stopped pulsating, the blood should flow out of cord into the baby. The cord will turn from blue to white. Tie a piece of sterile thread around it 15 cm (6 in) from baby's navel, then another at 20 cm (8 in). Check first tie is secure, or baby may lose blood. Sever cord between two ties with sterile scissors. Place a sterile dressing over the cut end. Leave for 10 minutes, then check there has been no bleeding. Tie a further thread 10 cm (4 in) from baby. Wash the mother.

BITES

Mammal bites: Danger from infection is the main risk. Anti-tetanus shots and rabies vaccine should be obtained before traveling. Rabies is untreatable without vaccine and almost always fatal. Symptoms: irritability, dislike of light, violent aversion to water and paralysis. Ensure the victim does not transmit the disease to anyone else.

Cleanse all bites, washing for at least 5 minutes to remove saliva. Then deal with bleeding, dress and bandage. Even if the bite heals, report it when you are rescued. You should be examined by a doctor.

Snake bites: Most species inject venom very deeply. Do not consider sucking or cutting the wound. To prevent poison spreading make the victim relax, apply pressure at the wound site and immobilize affected part. Apply a bandage—not a tourniquet— above the bite and bandage down over the bite (e.g., for an ankle bite, start bandaging at the knee). This should apply a firm pressure, but the limb should not darken or swell up. A splint will prevent flexing. If bite is on torso, apply pressure with wad of fabric. Place wound in cool water, e.g., a stream or use ice to cool. Try not to move the victim. Check pulse and breathing, stand by to give artificial respiration.

Spider bites: Treat as for snake bites. A cold compress helps reduce pain (ice wrapped in cloth is ideal).

Stings: Scorpions inject a powerful venom. Bee, wasp and hornet stings may cause severe allergic reactions, especially if there are multiple stings. Bee stings should be removed from the skin as quickly as possible by stroking sting with side of a needle, then extracting with tweezers. Do not squeeze the poison sac as this will release more venom. Apply a cold compress.

GENERAL POISONING

Do not induce vomiting—it can do more harm than good. It is only suitable if poisonous berries have very recently been swallowed: gently put a finger to the back of victim's throat. Never induce vomiting if corrosive substances, gasoline or solvents are involved.

Try to find out what has been swallowed. Burns around mouth indicate a caustic substance is involved. You must discover in advance the properties of chemicals to which you are exposed and appropriate remedies in cases of accident. Keep airway open: place victim in recovery position. Be prepared for vomiting, fits or convulsions. If breathing stops, give artificial respiration but avoid traces of poison around mouth.

Mix tea and charcoal—with milk of magnesia, if available. This antidote absorbs poison in the system.

Some plants, e.g., poison ivy, poison sumac and poison oak, cause skin irritation. Skin that has been in contact with the plant should be thoroughly washed with soap and water. Remove and wash clothing. Use alcohol to neutralize oil left on the skin.

> **☠ If handling a plant produces a severe reaction, do not put your hand to your face or touch other parts of the body until it has been well washed. Rashes and swellings can interfere with breathing, vision and urination.**

GENERAL DISORDERS

Small digestive upsets are relatively insignificant, but symptoms which suggest more serious conditions should not be ignored. If food is adequate the best treatment is to fast for a day and rest. Take plenty of fluids.

Treat fever with rest and aspirin, and find its causes.

More serious, pneumonia is indicated by inflammation of lungs with chills and fever, breathlessness, cough with green-yellow phlegm or blood, and pain in breathing. Keep the patient warm and give them frequent sips of hot water.

DISEASES

Infectious diseases are caused by bacteria (e.g., cholera, dysentery, tuberculosis), viruses (colds, flu, measles) and rickettsiae (e.g., typhus). Such contagious diseases are unlikely to occur unless you have brought them with you or catch them from humans you encounter.

The survivor is more likely to be exposed to waterborne diseases, or those carried by insects and animals. Tropical diseases are less familiar and will therefore be dealt with here in more detail. Where drugs are not available, treatment is largely a matter of dealing with symptoms and making patient comfortable.

Prevention is better than treatment. To avoid disease:

Get all suitable immunization before traveling

Purify drinking water

Clean hands when preparing or eating food

Wash and peel fruit

Sterilize eating utensils

Cover body to reduce risk of insect bites

Wash and smoke louse-ridden clothes

Wash body, but avoid swallowing water

Bury excreta

Protect food and drink from flies and vermin

Isolate outbreaks of infectious diseases. Keep contact with other members of group to minimum; boil all utensils used by the patient; cover cuts and sores against exposure to infection. Wash thoroughly after treating the patient. Avoid mucus from coughs and sneezes. Take special care disposing of patient's feces where they cannot spread infection or be disturbed.

> **Boil all water, even for cleaning teeth. Cover wounds and avoid standing in water in areas at risk.**

Worldwide diseases

Leptospirosis: Spread by rodents and infected water. Causes serious form of jaundice. Gains entry through cuts or sores, or in contaminated drinking water.
Symptoms: Jaundiced appearance, lethargy, fever.
Treatment: Procane penicillin and Tetracycline.

Infectious hepatitis: Passed on through infected feces or urine. Enters via contaminated water, and through cuts in skin.
Symptoms: Nausea, loss of appetite, abdominal pain. Skin usually turns yellowish.
Treatment: Rest and good nursing are the only treatment.

Poliomyelitis: Spread by contaminated drinking water.
Symptoms: Paralysis.
Treatment: Hot packs on muscles and good nursing.

Bacillary dysentery: Spread by flies, contaminated water and contact with feces containing the bacillus.
Symptoms: Blood-streaked feces, sudden high temperature.
Treatment: Antibiotics, rest, and plenty of fluids to counter risk of dehydration due to loss of body fluids.

Enteric (typhoid) fever: Caused by a salmonella bacillus.

Symptoms: Similar to dysentery, with headaches, abdominal pains, fever, loss of appetite, pains in limbs and delirium.

Treatment: Antibiotics. Inoculation will prevent it.

Cholera: A threat anywhere in unsanitary conditions.

Symptoms: Vomiting, loss of pulse at wrist, cold clammy skin and muscle cramps.

Protection: Can be obtained by regular inoculation with cholera vaccine.

WARM-CLIMATE DISEASES

Waterborne diseases

Bilharzia: Disease of bowel or bladder caused by microscopic worm endemic in parts of Africa, Arabia, China, Japan and S. America. Enters body through drinking infected water or through broken skin.

Symptoms: Irritation of urinary tract.

Treatment: Niridazole in recommended doses.

Hookworms: Gain entry through infected drinking water or penetrate bare skin (usually feet). Larvae may cause pneumonia. The worms live in the intestine.

Symptoms: Anemia and general lethargy.

Treatment: Alcapar and Mintazol in recommended doses. A decoction of bracken is a powerful de-wormer.

Amoebic dysentery: Transmitted in contaminated water and uncooked food.

Symptoms: Fatigue, listlessness. May produce a temperature. Feces may be solid but will smell foul and carry blood and jelly-like red mucus.

Treatment: Plenty of fluids, rest and treatment with Flagyl.

Insectborne diseases

To reduce risk keep skin covered, sleep under a mosquito net, use insect repellents, and do not camp near swamps or stagnant water. A course of tablets, begun before exposure, can protect against malaria.

Malaria: Not restricted to the tropics. Transmitted through saliva of female anopheles mosquito. It kills over a million people a year in Africa alone.

Symptoms: Recurrent fever. Although sweating, patient feels intensely chilled and shivers violently. There are various strains with severe headaches, malaise and vomiting accompanying the fever and leaving patient weak and exhausted.

Treatment: A number of anti-malarial drugs are available, including Larium, Paludrine, and now Malarone. Ask your doctor about which drug is most appropriate for your situation.

Dengue: Spread by mosquito.

Symptoms: Rash, headache, fever, extreme muscle and joint pains. Full recovery may take some weeks.

Treatment: Rest. There is no vaccine or cure.

Yellow fever: Prevalent in Africa, South America.

Symptoms: Headache, nosebleed, nausea and fever. Heartbeat may be slow. In severe cases: pain in legs, back and neck. Rapid liver damage may lead to jaundice and kidney failure.

Treatment: Rest and nursing. There is no effective drug. Obtain vaccination before traveling.

Typhus: A group of infectious diseases usually spread by insects such as fleas, mites and ticks.

Symptoms: Headache, constipation, collapse, back

pains and coughing, followed by fever, mild delirium, rash of small red spots. There may also be a weak heart-beat.

Treatment: *Antibiotics. There is also a vaccine available.*

> Small parasites which burrow beneath skin, e.g., larvae of warblefly, or the chigoe, should be removed before they can open up a route for further infection. Chigoes penetrate the skin of the feet or lower leg leaving red pinpricks in skin. Remove creatures with a needle and apply antiseptic ointment to the affected area.

WARM-CLIMATE AILMENTS

Prickly heat: Heavy sweating, coupled with rubbing by clothing, produces blockages in sweat glands.

Symptoms: Uncomfortable skin irritation.

Treatment: Remove clothing, wash body with cool water and put on dry clothes. Taking more liquid may make it worse. Antihistamine relieves discomfort.

Heat cramps: Often first warning of heat exhaustion.

Symptoms: Shallow breathing, vomiting, dizziness.

Treatment: Rest in shade. Drink water with a pinch of salt.

Heat exhaustion: Caused by exposure to heat and humidity. Can occur without direct exposure to sun.

Symptoms: Pale face, cold and clammy skin, weak pulse; with weakness, dizziness, and perhaps cramps. Delirium or unconsciousness may follow.

Treatment: As for cramps.

Heatstroke: The most serious result of heat exposure.

Symptoms: Hot dry skin; flushed, feverish face, but

sweating stops. Temperature rises, pulse rapid and strong. Severe headache, often with vomiting. Unconsciousness may follow.

Treatment: *Lay in shade, head and shoulders slightly raised. Remove outer clothing. Cool body by wetting underclothes with tepid (not cold) water and fanning. Do not fully immerse in water—sprinkle it over patient. Lay in well-ventilated hollow. When consciousness returns administer water to sip. When temperature returns to normal, replace clothing, keep warm.*

Immersion in cold water is very dangerous, but in extreme cases where risk of death or brain damage outweighs shock, use after initial cooling takes effect, lowering slowly into water. Massage extremities to increase blood flow. Remove from water as soon as temperature falls. Cover patient if it plummets. You may need to cool and cover several times before temperature stabilizes.

COLD-CLIMATE HAZARDS

Prolonged exposure to cold is dangerous anywhere.

Hypothermia: Loss of temperature due to exposure. Brought on by exhaustion, inadequate clothing or shelter, lack of food, lack of knowledge and preparation. Wet clothing or immersion in cold water will aggravate it, as will anxiety, stress, and injuries that immobilize.

Symptoms: *Irrational behavior: sudden bursts of energy followed by lethargy. Slowing of responses, sudden uncontrolled fits of shivering. Loss of coordination. Headaches, blurred vision and abdominal pains. Collapse or unconsciousness.*

Treatment: *Prevent further heat loss. Shelter from elements. Replace wet garments with dry, one item at a time. Apply warmth (other bodies, warm rocks). Place* *warmth in pit of stomach, small of back, armpits, back of neck, wrists, between thighs. Give warm fluids and sugary foods, but only if fully conscious. Do not administer alcohol. The patient is not cured when temperature returns to normal: recovery takes time.*

If heat is lost rapidly—rewarm rapidly
If heat is lost slowly—rewarm slowly

Frostbite: Occurs when skin and flesh freeze. Affects all exposed parts of the body and regions farthest from heart: hands, feet, face. First sign is often a prickly feeling, then waxy patches on skin which feel numb (later turning hard, pebbly, and painful, swelling, reddening and blistering before deadening and dropping off in final stage).

Prevention: Keep a constant lookout for signs: act at first appearance of waxy skin. Grimace to exercise face, flex hands, stamp feet. Never go out without adequate clothing. Avoid getting wet. Never touch metal with bare hands. Avoid spilling gasoline on bare flesh in sub-zero temperatures.

Treatment: Frostnip affects only the skin: warm the affected part (it will be painful when thawed). Deep frostbite should be gradually thawed with warm water at about the temperature which your elbow can comfortably bear. Do not rub with snow or expose to an open fire. Protect affected area from greater injury. Advanced frostbite may form blisters which can turn to ulcers. Do not burst blisters and never rub affected part. Use "animal warmth" to warm gradually; severe pain indicates it has been warmed too quickly.

Snow blindness: Temporary blindness. Can occur even in bright overcast periods with no direct sunlight.

Symptoms: Eyes become sensitive to glare; blinking

and squinting begins. Vision takes on pink/red hue. Eyes feel gritty.

Treatment: Get into dark place and blindfold eyes. Apply cool damp cloth to forehead. The condition is self-correcting.

Trench foot: Occurs when feet are immersed or are damp and cold for long periods. To prevent: keep feet dry, wear well-fitting boots, exercise feet and legs.

Symptoms: Pins and needles, then numbness interspersed with sharp pains. Feet appear purple with swelling and blisters.

Treatment: Dry the feet, but do not rub or damage blisters. Elevate feet and keep warm. Do not apply artificial heat. Do not massage. Rest and warmth are the cure.

NATURAL MEDICINE

Natural remedies can be used when medical supplies are exhausted, or to supplement your store. Urine can be used as an antiseptic to wash out wounds. Maggots will keep a wound open and clean until better treatment can be given (make sure they do not devour good tissues).

PLANT PREPARATIONS

Many modern drugs are derived from plants but the processes are complex, and attempts to use such plants in treatment could be very dangerous. What follows is a list of plants and medical uses to which they can be put in simple preparations. Identify plants carefully. As a general rule, plants are most potent when in flower. Different parts may have different uses. Larger or stronger doses may do more harm than good.

To make an infusion: Cut and crush herb, pour boiling water over, stir and leave to cool. No need to strain—

herbs will sink to bottom. If you can't boil water, use half the amount of cold and stand vessel in sun. Use a scant handful of herbs (30g/1g) to ½ liter (1 pint) water. If there is no sun or water, suck or chew leaves to extract the juices, then spit out the pulp.

To make a decoction: Cut, scrape and mash roots. Soak in water (handful to 85cc/1½ pints) for half hour. Bring to boil, simmer until liquid reduces by one third.

To make a poultice: Mash up roots, leaves or entire plant and make into a flat pad. Add water if too dry. Apply to affected part (stiff joints, sprains, abcesses) and cover with large leaf. Bind in position.

Expressed juice: Reduce stem and leaves to juicy mush by crushing with hands, rocks or sticks. Squeeze juice only into a wound and spread pulp around infected area. Keep in place with large leaf and bind.

REMEDIES
STOPPING BLEEDING:
Giant puffball: Packed as poultice
Plantain: Pounded leaves as poultice

CLEANSING RASHES/SORES/WOUNDS: Use externally
to bathe 2 or 3 times a day or, if indicated, as a poultice.
Burdock: Decoction of root; crushed raw root & salt for animal bites
Chickweed: Expressed juice of leaves
Comfrey: Decoction of root as poultice
Dead-nettle: Infusion of flowers and shoots
Dock: Crushed leaves
Elder: Expressed juice of leaves
Oak: Decoction of bark
Scurvey grass: Crushed leaves
Shepherd's purse: Infusion of whole plant, except roots, as poultice

Silverweed: Infusion of whole plant, except roots
Sorrel: Crushed leaves
Tansy: Crushed leaves
Watercress: Expressed juice

FEVERS: These plants will induce perspiration to break a fever.
   Elder: Infusion of flowers and fruit
   Lime: Infusion of flowers

ACHES/PAINS/BRUISES: Use externally where indicated.
   Birch: Infusion of leaves
   Borage: Infusion of whole plant, except roots
   Burdock: Decoction of root
   Chickweed: Infusion of whole plant, except roots
   Comfrey: Decoction of root applied to swellings
   Cowberry: Infusion of leaves and fruits
   Dock: Crushed leaves (bruises)
   Poplar: Infusion of leaf buds
   Sorrel: Crushed leaves applied to bruises
   Tansy: Crushed leaves applied to bruises
   Willow: Decoction of bark (headaches)

COLDS/SORE THROATS/RESPIRATORY COMPLAINTS:
   Angelica: Decoction of root
   Bilberry: Infusion of leaves and fruits
   Borage: Infusion of whole plant, except roots
   Burdock: Decoction of root
   Comfrey: Infusion of whole plant
   Horseradish: Raw root
   Lime: Infusion of flowers
   Nettle: Infusion of leaves
   Oak: Decoction of bark; use as gargle

Plantain: Infusion of leaves and stems
Poplar: Infusion of leaf buds
Rose: Decoction of hips
Willow: Decoction of bark

STOMACH UPSETS:

Bilberry: Decoction of fruit
Bracken: Infusion of leaves
Bramble: Infusion of leaves
Dandelion: Decoction of whole plant
Horseradish: Infusion of root
Mint: Infusion of whole plant, except root, with crushed charcoal

DIARRHEA: Take two or three times daily until symptoms subside.

Bilberry: Decoction of fruit
Bistort: Infusion of whole plant, except roots
Bramble: Infusion of leaves or decoction of fruit
Cowberry: Decoction of fruit
Great burnet: Infusion of leaves and shoots
Hazel: Infusion of leaves
Mint: Infusion of whole plant, except roots
Oak: Decoction of bark
Plantain: Infusion of leaves and stems
Silverweed: Infusion of whole plant, except roots

CONSTIPATION:

Barberry: Expressed juice of fruit
Couch grass (Elymus): Decoction of root
Dandelion: Decoction of whole plant
Elder: Expressed juice of fruit
Rowan: Expressed juice of fruit
Rose: Decoction of hips
Walnut: Decoction of bark

HEMORRHOIDS: Apply externally, 2 or 3 times a day.
Bilberry: Expressed juice of fruit
Oak: Decoction of bark
Plantain: Expressed juice
Poplar: Decoction of leaf buds
Silverweed: Infusion of whole plant, except roots

EXPELLING WORMS:
Bracken: Infusion of roots
Tansy: Infusion of leaves and flowers, use sparingly in small amounts

SOME USEFUL HERBAL PREPARATIONS

Headaches: Willow leaves and bark make a decoction containing salicin, a constituent of aspirin.

Healing: Expressed juice of comfrey leaves aids tissue regrowth.

Strawberry roots contain a descaler to clean teeth.

Delphinium seeds can be crushed to treat head lice.

Birch bark can be distilled to produce a tar oil which soothes skin complaints.

DISASTER
STRATEGIES

ACCIDENTS and isolation are not the only causes of a survival situation. Many natural and man-made forces can produce disasters in which your survival skills and strategies will come into play.

PREDICTING DISASTER
Meteorological stations around the world study weather conditions 24 hours a day and play a major role in warning of disasters. Monitor weather broadcasts for advance warning of severe weather conditions and disasters such as flooding, hurricanes, volcanic eruptions and earthquakes.

DROUGHT
In temperate regions, if rainfall drops far below the normal, periodic drought may be produced. The resulting death of vegetation causes deprivation right through the food chains that are based upon it. If the drought becomes severe, dead and dying animals may pollute what water supplies still remain.

Fire risk
Corpses of dead animals should be buried in deep graves. Dry ground can be very hard, but burying is the best way to remove these possible sources of infection.

The bodies could be burned, but since drought leaves everything tinder dry, a fire could easily get out of hand and, without water to check the flames, fire spreads rapidly. If you must have a fire, dig down to bare earth and keep the fire small and attended at all times.

Hygiene

Lack of water for washing and sanitation poses a health risk. Sweating will help to keep pores open and free of dirt, but, even when you need all available water for drinking, try to clean your hands after defecation and before preparing food. Make a latrine near the camp (see p. 139).

Store and conserve water

If a monsoon does not come, or a hot dry summer causes a parching of the earth, take precautions by storing as much water as possible and using it wisely. Keep it covered and shaded to avoid evaporation.

Dig a pit for a storage cistern in a shady spot, avoiding tree roots. Line it with a polythene sheet or with cement if available (but don't fill it up until the cement has had a chance to dry thoroughly). If there is clay in the area, dig a pit and line it with clay. If the clay or concrete is built into a partial dome, it will help to keep the contents cool and leave a smaller opening to keep covered.

 In conditions of severe drought be especially careful of contamination of water supplies. Disease from dead animals may be rampant. However thirsty you are, boil all water before drinking.

Never waste water. Water used for cooking can later be used for washing.

Boil all drinking water. If a well runs dry you may gain

more water by digging deeper, but the farther you dig, the more you deplete the water stored in the earth.

Try to eat foods with a high moisture content (such as fruit) and which require little preparation or clearing up afterward.

Flies may be a serious problem—ensure that all food-stuffs are covered. Protect your supplies from dust, which may become a hazard as top soil is blown away.

 When nature is disturbed by a severe drought, animals act abnormally. Crazed by thirst, normally docile creatures may attack you.

FIRE

The best protection from fire is prevention. Many fires are caused by carelessness with lighted cigarettes and burning matches. The sun shining through a piece of glass can start a blaze in a dry season.

FOREST FIRES

If you are present where a fire starts (or where a camp fire accidentally spreads) in woodland, or on heath or grass-land, your first action should be to smother it.

The first sign of an approaching forest fire will be the smell of smoke. Then you will probably hear the fire before you see flames. You may notice unusual animal behavior before you realize the cause.

Escape route

If caught in an area where fire is raging, and when it is far too late to put it out yourself, do not immediately flee—unless the fire is so close that there is no choice.

Even though you may feel that clothing hampers your movement, do not discard it for it will shield you from the full force of radiated heat.

Smoke will indicate the direction of the wind—the fire will be traveling fastest in that direction. If the wind is blowing away from you, toward the fire, move into the wind. Head for any natural fire break—such as a swathe through the trees, where the flames should be stopped. A river is the best break—even if the flames can leap it you will be reasonably safe in the water. In forestry plantations look for the firebreaks.

> Do not run wildly. Stop and think. Choose your escape route. Check the surrounding terrain and the wind direction to assess the possible spread of fire.

If the wind is blowing toward you the fire is likely to travel more quickly—and the flames can leap a larger gap. Fire travels faster uphill so do not make for high ground. Try to go around the fire if you can, but some forest fires burn on a front several kilometers wide, making it impossible. If you can neither skirt nor outdistance the blaze take refuge in a large clearing, deep ravine, watercourse or gully.

Going to earth

If you can semi-immerse yourself in a creek, so much the better. However, if there is no natural break or gully in which to shelter and the fire is too deep to think of running through, you may have to seek the protection of the earth itself.

People have survived fires by digging themselves in and covering themselves with earth, allowing the fire to burn over the top of them. The risk is great, not just from heat but from suffocation: fire burns up oxygen.

Scrape as much of a hollow as you can, clearing away grass and foliage, and throwing the earth on to a coat or cloth if you have one. Lie facedown and pull the cloth over you with its earth covering. Cup your hands over your mouth and nose and breathe through them. This won't increase the amount of oxygen, but it will cool down and filter the very hot air and sparks, which can damage the respiratory system. Try to hold your breath as the fire passes over.

STAY IN A VEHICLE

Don't try to drive through thick smoke. If caught in a fire in a vehicle, park in a clear area. Pull off the road, but don't risk getting bogged down. Turn on the headlights and stay inside the car. Wind windows tightly shut. Turn off the ventilation system and the seal air vents. The car will give you some protection from radiant heat. It is possible to survive by staying in a vehicle until the glass begins to melt, by which time the fire will have moved beyond you. There is a danger of a gasoline tank exploding but, if the fire is intense, your chances are much better inside the vehicle than outside.

Fighting a forest fire

In forestry plantations you should see racks of fire-beating equipment at intervals along the main routes. This consists of bundles of twigs, tied in a broom, and spade-shaped beaters with rubber blades. They can be effective in putting out the beginnings of a blaze.

Despite their name, do not beat rapidly with them. The object is to smother the fire by bringing the beater down over the flames to extinguish them.

If no equipment is available use a coat or blanket to smother the fire, or use a leafy branch to beat it out.

Fight fire with fire

Provided it is still some distance away, it may be possible to use fire to create protection when there is no way of getting out of the path of a forest fire or going through it.

The technique is to burn a patch of ground before the main fire reaches it. With nothing left to ignite, the flames cannot advance, giving you a place of refuge. The main fire must be sufficiently far away for your fire to burn a space it cannot jump before it arrives.

Light your own fire along as wide a line as possible, at least 10 m (30 ft) wide, but 100 m (300 ft) would be better. It will burn in the same direction as the main fire, creating a break which you can move into. Make sure you determine the wind direction correctly.

> BEWARE: Winds may be swirling and fires create their own drafts, so you may still have to make a dash through your own flames. The main fire must be far enough away for your own fire to burn and pass. Do not underestimate the speed at which flames travel— they may be approaching faster than you can run. Do not light another fire unless you are desperate and fairly certain of the outcome.

Escaping through fire

Sometimes the best escape route may be to run through the flames. This is impossible if they are very intense and the area covered by the fire is great. In a large clearing or on heath land, however, it may be possible to run through less dense fire to refuge on the already burned-out land.

Thick vegetation burns fiercely—so choose the spot for your breakthrough with care. Make your mind up, then do not delay. Dampen a piece of cloth to cover your nose and mouth. Cover as much exposed skin as you can (including your head) with a blanket, curtain or overcoat. If you have water available, tip some over you to damp down clothing, hair and any flesh you have not been able to cover. Take a deep breath. Cover your nose and mouth to keep out smoke and run.

If your clothes catch alight do not stay on your feet when out of the fire. Flames and smoke will travel up your body, over your face and into your lungs.

> Do not run if your clothes are ablaze—this will only fan the flames. Roll on the ground and try to wrap yourself in something that will smother the flames—a mat, blanket or overcoat.

If someone else comes running out of a fire with their clothes alight, push them to the ground and use the same methods of denying the flames oxygen. Do not hug them to you, or your clothes may catch fire.

FIRES IN BUILDINGS

Block gaps around doors and windows. Close all blinds and curtains. Stay away from outside walls and don't be panicked into running out of the house when the fire reaches it.

Once the fire has passed, avoid excessive smoke inhalation, but go outside and put out any small fires.

VEHICLE FIRES

The greatest danger with cars is the risk of the fuel tank being ignited. The aim is to control the fire before it can reach the tank. Everything has a flash point and a fuel tank is more at risk than most things. Usually a fuel line (if not armored) will catch fire first, acting as a fuse which eventually ignites the tank.

If a car catches fire in a confined space, smoke and toxic fumes will soon build up. Try to put the fire out first—but if that is not practicable remove the car from the building before it further endangers life and property. Do not get into the car. You can do everything from outside, including steering. If possible, push or pull the car out. If your car has a starter button, select a low gear or reverse and use the starter to bounce the car out. With conventional ignition, turn the key in short bursts. Be prepared for the car to jerk forward violently.

In a crashed car doors may jam. If it catches fire get through any window or kick the windscreen out. If the fire is inside the car use the extinguisher or smother it with a rug or coat. Synthetic materials used in upholstery in many cars burn rapidly and give off thick smoke and toxic gases. These will persist even when the flames are extinguished, so get out into the air as soon as possible.

KEEP YOUR FIRE EXTINGUISHER HANDY!
Don't keep your fire extinguisher in the boot or trunk—keep it where you can get at it immediately. Impact could distort the boot lid and prevent your opening it.

FIRES IN THE AIR

Airplanes are equipped with automatic extinguishers for engine fires and handheld extinguishers in the cabin. Action should be taken immediately. On civil airlines summon a flight attendant immediately you suspect fire—the staff know where equipment is and how to use it. Avoid creating panic among other passengers. If you see smoldering or flames, smother with an airline blanket or clothing.

The main fire dangers are before take-off when there is volatile fuel and vapor around the plane, and especially when landing under difficult circumstances when fuel tanks could be ruptured and electrical or friction sparks ignite aviation spirit. Every safety precaution is taken to ensure that fire is not a hazard. You can help. Do not smoke, when told not to smoke. Do not smoke and doze at the same time.

FLOOD

Flooding can occur for many reasons. It may be caused by the overflowing of rivers, lakes and reservoirs caused by heavy rains (not necessarily rainfall at the place where the flood occurs); by the buildup of sea or lake water due to the effects of submarine earthquake, hurricanes and freak high tides and winds; or by the collapse of dams or dikes.

Heavy rain can rapidly produce torrents where there was a dry riverbed, or a buildup in a narrow channel or behind a barrier which then gives way to a rushing wall of water that envelops everything in its path.

Persistent rainfall over a long period after a dry spell and heavy storms should alert you to keep clear of water channels and low-lying ground, but a flood can affect much wider areas. It is always safer to camp on a spur. If the water is rising, move to higher ground. In hilly areas keep out of valley bottoms, which are particularly prone to flash floods.

Food is not likely to be a problem, at least at first, for animals will also head for high ground. Both predators and prey are likely to concentrate on getting to safety—but beware of injury from panic-stricken animals in the water.

Drinking water may be difficult to obtain, for the water swirling around you may be contaminated. Collect rainwater to drink, and boil any other water before you use it.

Flooded buildings

If you are in a building when the water begins to rise, stay where you are. You will be less at risk than trying to evacuate on foot. Turn off gas and electricity and prepare emergency food supplies, warm clothing and drinking water in well-sealed containers. Collect a torch, whistle, mirror and brightly colored cloths for signaling, and add them to your gear with a camp stove, candles, and matches.

Move to an upper floor, or on to the roof in a single-story building. If you are forced to occupy the roof, erect a shelter. If it is a sloping roof, tie everyone to a chimney stack or other solid structure. If the water continues to rise, prepare some kind of raft. If you have no ropes, use bed sheets. Unless the water rises so high you are forced to evacuate, stay until it stops rising.

Evacuation

Seek shelter on higher ground. You don't have to be at the bottom of a hill to be on low ground!

When walking or driving to a safer location remember that a small drop in the level of the roadway down a hill can make a difference to the water depth.

If your car stalls, abandon it. You and your vehicle could be swept away.

Do not attempt to cross a pool or a stream unless you are certain the water will not be higher than the center of the car's wheels or your knees. If you must cross, use the river-crossing techniques explained on pp. 191–195. If crossing bridges which are under water take special care if flood has already swept part of the bridge away.

Flash floods

In a sudden heavy rainfall keep out of valley bottoms and streambeds both during and after rainfall. You don't have to be at the bottom of a hill to be caught by water rushing down it carrying mud and debris.

Coastal flooding

This is usually a combination of high tides and winds which make them even higher. Flood warnings will usually be given and evacuation is the best action.

Flood aftermath

Do not go outside until you know it's safe. More storms could be on the way.

As flood waters recede they leave a scene of devastation littered with debris and the bodies of flood victims. With decay and the pollution of the water comes the risk of disease. Take extra precautions: burn all animal corpses—do not risk eating them—and thoroughly boil all water before using. Some crops may still be available after the flood waters recede and birds that have escaped the flood will be safe and good to eat.

TSUNAMI

A tsunami, or tidal wave, is linked with an earthquake beneath the ocean, creating a series of waves which can reach more than 30 m (100 ft) high and travel vast distances causing damage along coasts. Not all earthquakes cause tsunami, but any earthquake could.

Keep away from shores and take to higher ground when there are tremors. Do not go to look for a tsunami—if you are close enough to see one, you are too close to escape it, unless high above its level. There is no defense against a moving wall of water. Evacuate.

A tsunami is not one wave but a series. Do not return to the danger area after the first wave as you may be killed by the onslaught of a second or third.

AVALANCHE

There are several types of avalanche.

SOFT-SLAB AVALANCHE

Snow falling on lee slopes, often below a cornice, fails to settle and compact like the snow below. A gap forms behind. It may feel hard and safe but any disturbance or loud noise can set the whole slab in motion.

AIRBORNE AVALANCHE

Frequently the result of new snow falling on an already

hard crust or in cold, dry conditions. This may begin as a slab avalanche, but gathers momentum and more powdered snow to reach very high speeds. Cover nose and mouth to stand a chance of survival—death is caused by drowning from inhaling snow.

WET-SNOW AVALANCHE

More common in times of thaw, often following a rapid temperature rise after snowfall. It moves more slowly than an airborne avalanche, picking up trees and rocks in its path. When it stops it freezes solid almost instantly, making rescue very difficult.

Lay flat and use crawl stroke to keep on top of slide (the debris can form a very deep layer). Get rid of pack and other encumbrances. Cover nose and mouth to avoid swallowing snow. When you come to rest, make as big a cavity around you as you can before the snow freezes, and try to reach the surface. Slip off any kit you have not been able to discard—it will hamper your extraction. Save your energy to shout when you hear people.

HURRICANE

A hurricane is a wind of high speed—above force 12 on the Beaufort Scale—which brings torrential rain and can destroy any flimsy structures. It is a tropical form of cyclone, which in more temperate latitudes would be prevented from developing in the upper levels of the air by the prevailing westerly winds.

> **Hurricanes are known by various names around the world:**
> **Hurricane: Caribbean and North Atlantic, eastern North Pacific, western South Pacific.**
> **Cyclone: Arabian Sea, Bay of Bengal, southern Indian Ocean.**

Typhoon: China Sea, western North Pacific.
Willy-willy: Northwest Australia.

Hurricanes develop over the ocean when sea temperatures are at their highest, especially in late summer. Warm air creates a low pressure core around which winds may rotate at speeds up to 300 kph (200 mph) or more, circling anticlockwise in the northern hemisphere, clockwise in the southern. The strongest winds are usually 16–19 km (10–12 miles) from the center of the hurricane but the center, or eye, brings temporary calm. The eye may be up to 500 km (300 miles) in diameter. Hurricanes can occur at any time of year: in the northern hemisphere, the main season is June to November, and in the southern, November to April (especially January and February). Hurricanes are not a feature of the South Atlantic.

Pattern of the hurricane

Out at sea hurricanes will build up force and begin to veer toward the Pole, the wind speed usually being greatest on the poleward side of the eye.

Hurricane warnings

Satellite surveillance enables meteorologists to track hurricanes and to warn of their approach. Some move very erratically, so monitor forecasts in hurricane areas.

Without radio to alert you, the growth of swell can indicate a hurricane, especially when coupled with other conditions such as highly colored sunsets or sunrises; dense banners of cirrus cloud converging toward the vortex of the approaching storm; and abnormal rises in barometric pressure followed by an equally rapid drop.

PRECAUTIONS
Get out of the hurricane's path if you can. Hurricane warnings

are usually issued when one is expected within 24 hours and will give you plenty of time to evacuate its path, if you are prepared.

Keep away from the coast and from riverbanks.

Board up windows and secure any objects outdoors that might be blown away.

At sea take down canvas, batten down hatches and stow all gear.

If you are in a solid building and on high ground stay where you are—travel in a hurricane is extremely dangerous. The safest place is usually in a cellar or under the stairs. Do not shelter near an internal chimney breast—the chimney may collapse.

Store drinking water—water and power supplies may be cut off by the storm—and have a battery-operated radio to listen for any instructions.

If you are not in a sturdy structure, evacuate to a hurricane shelter. Shut off power supplies before you leave.

Do not drive in a hurricane. Cars offer no protection from high winds and flying debris.

Seeking shelter

Outdoors, a cave will offer the best protection. A ditch will be next best. If unable to escape, lie flat on the ground where you will be less of a target for flying debris. Crawl to the leeside of any really solid shelter such as a stable rocky outcrop or a wide belt of large trees. Beware of small trees and fences which could be uprooted.

Stay where you are when the hurricane appears to have passed—there will usually be less than an hour of calm

as the eye passes and then the winds will resume in the opposite direction. If sheltering outdoors move to the other side of your windbreak in preparation or move to better shelter if close by.

TORNADO

Tornadoes are the most violent of atmospheric phenomena and the most destructive over a small area. Wind speeds have been estimated at 620 kph (400 mph).

The diameter of the twister at ground level is usually only 25–50 m (80 ft) but, within it, the destruction is enormous. Everything in its path except the most solid structures is sucked up into the air. The difference in pressure outside and inside a building is often the cause of collapse. Tornadoes can sound like a spinning top or engine and have been heard up to 40 km (25 miles) away. They travel at 50–65 kph (30–40 mph).

TORNADO PRECAUTIONS

Take shelter in the most solid structure available, ideally in a storm cellar or cave. In a cellar stay close to an outside wall, or in a specially reinforced section. If there is no basement, go to the center of the lowest floor, into a small room or shelter under sturdy furniture—but not where there is heavy furniture on the floor above. Keep well away from windows.

Close all doors and windows on the side facing the oncoming whirlwind and open those on the opposite side. This will prevent the wind getting in and lifting the roof as it approaches, and equalize the pressure to prevent the house "exploding."

Do not stay in a caravan or car, it could be drawn up in the storm. Outdoors you are vulnerable to flying debris and to being lifted up. You can see and hear a tornado coming. Get out of the way. Move at right angles to its apparent path. Take shelter in a ditch or depression, lie flat and cover your head with your arms.

LIGHTNING

Lightning can be especially dangerous on high ground or when you are the tallest object. In a lightning storm keep away from hill brows, from tall trees and lone boulders. Make for low, level ground and lie flat.

Insulation

If you cannot get away from tall objects, sit on dry material, which will provide insulation. A dry coil of climbing rope makes good insulation. Do not sit on anything wet. Bend your head down and hug your knees to your chest, lifting your feet off the ground and drawing in all your extremities. Do not reach down to the ground with your hands, that could give a contact to conduct the lightning. If you have nothing which will insulate you from the ground lie as flat as you can.

Stay low

You can sometimes sense that a lightning strike is imminent by a tingling in the skin and the sensation of the hair standing up on end. If you are standing up, drop to the ground at once, going first to the knees with the hands touching the ground. If you should be stuck, the charge may take the easiest route to the earth through your arms—missing the torso and possibly saving you from heart failure or asphyxiation. *Quickly lie flat.*

Do not hold metal objects when there is lightning about and keep away from metal structures and fences. However, do not jettison equipment if you will lose it altogether (when climbing, for instance). A dry axe with a wooden handle may spark at the tip, but is well insulated.

Proximity to large metal objects can be dangerous,

even without contact, for the shockwave caused by the heated air—as the lightning passes—can cause damage to the lungs.

Shelter

One of the best places to shelter in a lightning storm is at least 3 m (10 ft) inside a deep cave with a minimum of 1 m (4 ft) space on either side of you.

Do not shelter in a cave mouth or under an overhang of rock in mountainous country. Lightning can spark across the gap. Small openings in the rock are frequently the ends of fissures which are also drainage routes and automatic lightning channels.

EARTHQUAKE

Earthquakes come suddenly with little warning. Minor earth tremors can happen anywhere, but major quakes are confined to known earthquake belts.

With monitoring by seismologists, earthquakes can be predicted and evacuation may be possible. Animals become very alert, tense and ready to run.

A succession of preliminary tremors, known as fore-shocks, often followed by a seismically quiet period, usually precede a major quake, which they can actually trigger. These initial tremors may not be noticeable.

DOMESTIC EARTHQUAKE PRECAUTIONS

Stay tuned to a local radio station for up-to-date reports and advice if you have warning of a possible earthquake.

Turn off gas, electricity and water if advised to do so.

Remove large and heavy objects from high shelves.

Have ready in case needed: fresh water and emergency food, a torch, first-aid materials and a fire extinguisher.

EARTHQUAKE PRECAUTIONS

In a building

Stay indoors. Douse fires. Stay away from glass, including mirrors, and especially from large windows. An inside corner of the house, or a well-supported interior doorway are good places to shelter. A lower floor or a cellar gives the best chance of survival. Make sure there are plenty of exits. Get under a table or large piece of furniture, which will give both protection and an air space. In a shop keep away from large displays of goods. In high-rise offices never go into an elevator. Staircases may attract panicking people. Get under a desk.

In a car

Stop as quickly as you can, but stay in the car—it will offer some protection from falling objects. Crouch down below seat level and you will be further protected if anything falls on the car. When the tremors cease keep a watch for any obstructions and hazards such as broken cables and undermined roadways or bridges which could give way.

Outdoors

Lie flat on the ground. Do not try to run. You will be thrown about and could be swallowed in a fissure. Keep away from tall buildings and trees. Do not deliberately go underground or into a tunnel where you could be trapped by collapse. If you have managed to get to an open space do not move back into buildings for if minor tremors follow they could collapse any structure left unstable by the first quake.

On a hillside it is safer to get to the top. Slopes are liable to landslide and there would be little chance of survival. People have been known to survive by rolling into a tight ball on the ground.

Beaches—provided they are not below cliffs—are initially fairly safe but, since tidal waves often follow a quake you should move off the beach to high open ground as soon as the tremor has finished. Further tremors are unlikely to be as dangerous as a tsunami.

Be calm and think fast: speed is essential if an earthquake strikes. There is little time to organize others. Use force if necessary to get them to safety or pull them to the ground.

AFTER THE EARTHQUAKE

Check yourself and others for injuries. Apply first aid if necessary.

Rupture of sewage systems, contamination of water and the hazards of the bodies trapped in the wreckage can all make the risk of disease as deadly as the earthquake itself. Bury all corpses, animal and human. Take special precautions over sanitation and personal hygiene. Filter and boil all water. Check that sewage services are intact before using lavatories.

Do not shelter in damaged buildings or ruins. Build a shelter from debris. Be prepared for aftershocks. Open cupboards carefully, objects may tumble out. Clean up spilled household chemicals and potentially harmful substances. Do not strike matches or lighters, or use electrical appliances, if there is any chance of a gas leak. Sparks ignite gas.

VOLCANO

Active volcanoes are found in the areas of the world which are also most prone to earthquakes.

ERUPTION HAZARDS

Although it is possible to outrun most basalt lava flows they continue relentlessly until they reach a valley bottom or eventually cool off. They crush and bury anything in their path. Lava flows are probably the least hazard to life, for the able-bodied can escape them. Other hazards are more dangerous.

Missiles

Volcanic missiles, ranging from pebble-size fragments to lumps of rock and hot lava, can be scattered over vast distances. Volcanic ash can cover an even greater area.

If evacuating from close to the volcano, hard helmets offer some protection. Over a wider area, evacuation may not be necessary, but protection should be worn against the ash and any accompanying rain.

Ash

Volcanic ash is pulverized rock forced out in a cloud of steam and gases. Abrasive, irritant and heavy, its weight can cause roofs to collapse. It smothers crops, blocks transport routes and watercourses and, combined with toxic gases, can cause lung damage to the very young, the old and those with respiratory problems. Only very close to an eruption are gases concentrated enough to poison healthy people. However, when ash is combined with rain, sulphuric acid (and other acids) are produced in concentrations which can burn skin, eyes and mucous membranes. Wear goggles which seal the area around the eyes (not sunglasses, which will offer no protection). Use a damp cloth over the mouth and nose, or, better still, industrial dust masks. On reaching shelter remove clothing, thoroughly wash exposed skin and flush eyes with clean water.

Gas balls

A ball of red-hot gas and dust may roll down the side of a volcano at speeds of more than 160 kph (100 mph).

Unless there is an underground shelter nearby, the only chance of survival is to submerge under water and hold your breath for the half-minute or so it will take to pass.

Mud flows

The volcano may melt ice and snow and cause a glacial flood or—combined with earth—create a mud flow, known as a lahar. This can move at up to 100 kph (60 mph) with devastating effect. In a narrow valley a lahar can be as much as 30 m (100 ft) high. They are a danger long after the major eruption is over and are a risk even when the volcano is dormant if it generates enough heat to produce meltwater retained by ice barriers. Heavy rains may cause it to breach the ice.

Volcanoes usually show increased activity before a major eruption. Sulphurous smells from rivers, stinging acidic rain, loud rumblings or plumes of steam from the volcano are all warning signs.

Remember if evacuating by that car: ash may make roads slippery, even if it does not block them. Avoid valley routes which could become the path of the lahar.

VEHICLES

Transport has an important role to play in disaster strategy. Make sure you know how to get the best use out of your vehicle in any situation.

BEFORE SETTING OFF

For desert travel, fit long-range fuel tanks and make provision for storing drinking water. Carry further supplies of both in jerry cans. A jack is no use in soft sand and an air bag should be carried, which is inflated by the exhaust. Extra filters will be needed in the fuel line and air intake. Sand tires must be fitted and sand channels carried to get you moving again when bogged down in loose sands.

For high altitudes adjust the carburetor. In scrub country, thorn gaiters will reduce puncture risks. Antifreeze and suitable wheels and chains are needed for snow and ice. The engine will need special tuning to match climatic conditions and its own spares. Carry a spare wheel and a good tool kit.

IN HOT CLIMATES

Overheating: Stop and allow the engine to cool. If you are driving a particularly tricky stretch and stopping is out of the question, switch on the heater. This will give greater volume to the cooling water and, although the inside of the car will get even hotter, the engine will cool. When convenient stop and open up the hood. Do not undo the radiator cap until the temperature drops. Check the radiator and all hoses for leaks. If the radiator is leaking, adding the white of an egg will seal small holes. If there is a large hole, squeeze the section of the copper piping flat to seal it off. It will reduce the size of the cooling area but, if you drive very steadily, you will be able to keep going.

Metal gets hot: Be careful! All metal parts of a car can become hot enough to cause blisters.

 Never leave an injured person or an animal in a closed car in a hot climate—or even on a sunny day in temperate regions. Always leave windows open to ensure ventilation. Heat exhaustion kills even in the shade, as the sun will move.

Care in sandy conditions: When adding fuel, sand and dust can get into the tank. Rig a filter over or just inside the inlet to the tank.

IN COLD CLIMATES

If you are trapped in a blizzard, stay in the car. If you are on a regular traffic route you will probably soon be rescued. Going for help could be too risky.

Run the engine for heat if you have fuel. Cover the engine so that as little heat as possible is lost, but make sure the exhaust is clear. Do not risk exhaust fumes coming into the car. If you feel drowsy stop the engine and open a window. Do not go to sleep with the engine running. Switch off the heater as soon as you have taken the chill off, starting it again when temperature drops. If there is no fuel, wrap up in any spare clothing, rugs, etc. and keep moving inside the car.

If you have to leave the car to go a short distance, e.g., if you know help is very close, rig up a signpost—a bright scarf on a stick will help you find the car again.

When the blizzard stops, if it is daylight (otherwise wait until morning), it is worth walking out if there is a clear guide to the route (such as telegraph poles).

If miles from anywhere and the snow is building up to bury the car, get out and build yourself a snow cave. When the blizzard stops scrape large signs in the snow and use other signals to attract attention.

Starting: Always try to park on a gradient so that you can use a bump start to back up the starter. Once you get the engine going keep it running, but check that the handbrake is firmly on and never leave children or animals in an unattended vehicle with the engine running.

Demisting: Don't try to drive looking through a small clear patch on a misty screen. Rub onion or raw potato on the inside of the screen to stop it misting up.

Cover the outside of windscreen and windows with newspaper to prevent frost building up on them. If damp, however, paper will stick.

Cover the engine: Wrap a blanket around the engine to help stop it from freezing up, but remember to remove it before you start the engine. Cover lower part of the radiator with cardboard or wood so that it does not freeze as you go along. If very cold, leave covered. Otherwise remove to prevent overheating.

Cover metal: Don't touch any metal with bare hands. Your fingers could freeze to it and tear off skin. Where handling metal components with gloves is awkward, wrap fingers with adhesive tape. Treat radiator cap and dip stick in this way to ease your daily checks.

Diesel engines: Diesel contains water and freezes solid at low temperatures. Always cover front of engine, but check for overheating. Wrap engine at night or when left standing. Some drivers light small fires under frozen tanks. Only you can judge if the risk is worth taking.

GENERAL

Clutch slip: Often caused by oil or grease getting on the clutch plates. To degrease, use the fire extinguisher. Squirt it through inspection plate opening.

Broken fan belt: Improvise with tights, a tie or string.

High tension leads: If a high tension lead breaks, you may be able to replace it with a willow twig. Any plant stem with water content will carry current from the coil to distributor. Spit on ends and insert them into push-fit contacts. When you switch on, there is a deadly current of about 1300 volts: do not touch. Replace the twig frequently as it dries out.

Dead battery: Set the vehicle moving by a tow, a push or letting it run downhill. Select second gear and release the clutch to bump start.

CREDITS AND ACKNOWLEDGMENTS

This book was edited and designed by
Anne O'Brien and Stephen Kirk

Other illustrations were drawn by
Steve Cross, Chris Lyon,
Andrew Mawson, Tony Spalding

The editors would also like to thank
the following for their assistance:
Belinda Bouchard, Ronald Clark, Mark Crean,
Johnny Pinfold, William Spalding

Department of Community Affairs,
State of Florida, USA

Department of Emergency Management,
State of Washington, USA

Federal Emergency Management Agency,
Washington, DC, USA

Greater London Council Fire Brigade Department, UK

Health and Safety Commission, UK

Office of Emergency Services,
State of California, USA